MW00680089

A Cure for Emma

One Mother's Journey to Oz

Julie Colvin

www.acureforemma.com

Praise for *"A Cure for Emma"* by Julie Colvin

"From one *Mother Warrior* to another, I have deep respect and compassion for Julie's brave and loving journey in search of a cure for her daughter. Nothing is more powerful than mommy intuition and perseverance as one travels down this difficult, uncharted road. I commend Julie for her tenacity and dedication. You go girl! Much love and best wishes with your journey and your book."

~ Jenny McCarthy ~
comedian, actress, model, author, activist

"Nothing touches us more meaningfully than the story of a parent's care for a child-in-need. As the father of a diabetic, I understand Julie's roller coaster of despair, frustration, and hope. The love we feel for our kids is unlike any other emotion in the human spectrum, and capturing it in prose is an art. With gratitude and congratulations to Julie."

~ Alan Thicke ~
actor, songwriter, game-and talk-show host

"Thank you, Julie, for your contribution toward our shared goal of finding a cure for our children. I wish you much success with your book *A Cure for Emma*, and look forward to the day all T1 families can celebrate the successful outcome of this goal."

~ Denise Jonas ~
mother of Nick Jonas
singer, songwriter, musician and actor

"The Faustman Lab is proud to support Julie Colvin and her ongoing efforts to raise awareness about type 1 diabetes. This disease demands constant vigilance and determination on the part of diabetics and their families. Our hope is this book will shed light on the issues surrounding this disease, and facilitate the advancement of a cure."

~ Dr. Denise Faustman ~
Director Immunobiology Laboratory,
Associate Professor of Medicine, Harvard Medical School

"I cried. I laughed. I didn't want the ride to end. This book blows the dust off our hearts, showing us how to see our past with more clarity and move forward with renewed faith and purpose. Truly a life-transforming, courageous, and inspiring journey."

~ Linda Sivertsen ~

award-winning author, magazine editor,
NYT bestselling co-author, and environmentalist.

Copyright © 2011 by Julie Colvin

NorLightsPress.com
762 State Road 458
Bedford IN 47421

All rights reserved. No part of this book may be reproduced or transmitted in any form or by any means, electronic or mechanical, including photocopying, recording or by any information storage and retrieval system, without written permission from the author, except for the inclusion of brief quotations in a review.

Printed in the United States of America
ISBN: 978-1-935254-52-2

Cover design concept by Wendy Janssen
Book design by Nadene Carter

First printing, 2011

PUBLISHER'S NOTE: The medical and health information discussed in this book is not intended to replace the services of trained health professionals or be a substitute for medical advice. You are advised to consult with your health care professional with regard to matters relating to your health, and in particular regarding matters that may require diagnosis or medical attention.

For my children:
May you always know how incredible you are!

Acknowledgements

This book is a work of nonfiction. I have changed or omitted some names of friends and family to protect their privacy and have identified these occasions throughout the story.

The words on the following pages were born from a place of love, faith, and gratitude: love for my children, Emma and Will, who mean more to me than my humble words can ever describe. And love for my husband, Marc – my lighthouse on the stormy shore – the one person whose friendship, dedication, and tolerance of my spiritual wanderings enabled me to follow this whimsical, intuitive, and grandiose idea – to actually write a book. Who knew?

Thank you to my leading ladies and to all the incredible people who have come into my life: my friends, my teachers, my soul sisters (you know who you are). I would have nothing to write about if it weren't for you. You taught me there are no boundaries to support and acceptance. We are truly all connected heart to heart, and for this I will be eternally grateful.

Thank you to Dr. P. J. Pace, the best family physician anyone could ask for, and to his irreplaceable secretary Peggy for coming into our lives shortly after Emma's diagnosis. This was a critical time for our family and your compassionate medical shoulder was an excellent place to lean while we found our balance. Equal thanks go out to our diabetes team at the Hospital for Sick Children in Toronto. Such a gift to have access to some of the best diabetes care, in the world!

Thank you to my **L** angels. I used your beautiful names as my leading lady aliases. You are the most incredible women I will ever know, and your support and guidance enabled me to pull off this herculean endeavor:

L 1. **L**ois Weston-Bernstein – my BFF and personal blog editorial advisor. You are blessed with literary eyes as sharp as an eagle and a well-earned reputation for being clever enough to land a space shuttle with a calculator. You're amazing.

L 2. **L**eila Summers – my fellow writer's workshop companion and instigator of all things internet. Your countless late night hours helping me establish an online presence is perhaps the single strongest reason I didn't put my scribbles in a desk drawer to be looked at when I'm old and grey. Putting my intentions out into the world committed me to my goal – to write this book. For this I have you, and you alone, to thank.

L 3. **L**isa Fugard – my writing coach. Thank you for gently steering me through multiple drafts. Your guidance to help me build my story as a compelling narrative was invaluable to my journey and to this book. Hay House publishing is truly blessed to have you as their writing workshop instructor, and I'm truly blessed to have met you.

L 4. **L**inda Sivertsen – my guru and mentor extraordinaire. I have only the universe to thank for getting us together in Carmel, and the rest is history. Your friendship, guidance, and mad writing skills, along with blueprints on how to write a winning book proposal, were the defining moments for this project. You are an incredible support to writers everywhere and one of the finest women I know. www.winningbookproposals.com

I reserve the biggest thank you of all for my agent Krista Goering and the publishing team at Norlights Press for believing in me and my work. I am forever grateful for the opportunity you have given me.

Finally, I must shout out to all my Facebook peeps. I'm blessed to be a part of this incredible global online community. What exciting times we live in, to have this opportunity to connect. I am also deeply honored to host the *T1 Diabetes Cure – Global Headquarters* Facebook page, with posts from leading research organizations and scientists in the world. This online multinational tribe of T1 warriors has been my largest source of inspiration. *A Cure for Emma* is for all of us. Together we *are* bringing the T1 cure into our lives!

Table of Contents

Introduction

I CLOSE MY EYES AND LET MY FINGERS fly across the keys until I feel clear again, my thoughts quieting. Patterns begin to reveal themselves within the silent spaces between the words. I keep digging, keep writing – hoping to regain a sense of balance. My motivation for this new obsession? To find my north star in the cloudy night sky. To become healthy and happy once again. And above all to find a cure for my daughter, Emma.

First Journal Entry, March 2007 ~ Inspired by a Dream

I'm no one special.

I'm a good mother, wife, and friend, but not extraordinary in any way. I've often dreamed about making a difference, doing something special, even saving the world. But how?

I've wondered about this since I was young. Over the years I caught glimpses of the spiritual path, yet was easily distracted as life flowed around me. Unaware of my ability to control the journey, sometimes I felt exhilarated and invincible; at other times I felt beaten down and unworthy.

When I look at people who do amazing things, I'm humbled. If only I could wipe the tears from children's faces in distant countries, stop the injustice of war, or cure disease. But how could *I* make a difference – one tiny speck of energy in this overwhelming cosmos?

Today, my perception is shifting as I begin to awaken; a wake-up call provided by an *incurable disease* lurking within my precious daughter. A disease that, through its wily wisdom, introduces me to a place of simplicity, like jumping into an ice-cold sea of awareness:

I AM the sea.

I AM the crying child.

I AM the injustices of war.

If I want my daughter to be free of the burdens that challenge her daily existence, I must be willing to break free of the baggage that challenges mine.

I will focus on nurturing myself and choose to believe in the possibilities of my life. I will feed my body, mind, and spirit with caring, open thoughts. This will touch the people I love and flow like a wave to the rest of the universe.

When I do this, the path becomes open for my children to do the same. The path becomes open for all the world. Imagine what it could be like: No weapons used against one another; no harm done to our beautiful planet; no illness to take away the gift of health or life before one's time. Only compassion and love for all, because that is what we feel for ourselves.

I may be no one special, *but I can save the world.*

Part 1

Contrast Brings Clarity

As we live the darkest depths of our fears,
we see more clearly the heights of our desires.

Chapter 1

The Land of Oz

June 2007

SUNLIGHT FILTERS THROUGH the narrow slats of my shades and I turn to check the time – 6:30 a.m. I don't need to be up for another thirty minutes, but I've awakened early today. I roll over, hoping to fall back to sleep – God knows I could use more of that – when I notice it again. Something soft and fluffy tickles my toes.

I move my feet to probe the curious object beneath the sheets. Perhaps one of my children's stuffed animals has gone MIA, or I'm still asleep and dreaming. *Youch!* Definitely not sleeping. Sharp kitten teeth sink into my big toe.

Mojo, our treasured black fluff of fur has crawled beneath the blankets, chasing my toes like a proud hunter. She's too adorable to be irritating. I reach to find her chubby kitten belly and lift her to my lips for a counter-attack of good morning kisses.

~ ~ ~ ~

Tender memories wash over me as I breathe in this deeply familiar feeling. She reminds me of my childhood pet, Puss 'n Boots.

When I was six years old, Boots would curl around my feet and keep them warm during cold winter nights. Most of my childhood memories are filled with upheaval and uncertainty, so I try not to dwell on that part of my life. This morning, however, bits and pieces come flitting in.

We had Boots during the times I lived with my mom. In the middle of never knowing where we might live next, our kitty was the one thing I could count on to bring me to a happy place. Like a direct link to goodness and security, my cat offered a guaranteed state of bliss.

I call up a few other rare, fond memories: fun-filled times when my older sister and I visited my dad's parents in their log cottage two hours north of Toronto. I cherished those weekends of dress-up fun, laughing as we played on the beach and chased Harvey, the wild, friendly bunny through the trees. Most of all, I loved fishing with Grandpa.

As for my mother's parents, my sister and I lived with them for a year when I was in grade two. I spent hours in the lush woods and meadows around their century-old farmhouse with its majestic barn and enticing chicken coop. Strolling through the dew covered grass to collect warm eggs each morning was a highlight for anyone who visited.

We called our grandma Chicken Grammy. She provided structure and routine during that year, including regular healthy meals, guitar lessons on the front patio, and involvement with school activities to keep us active. What I remember most was her magnificent and glorious color TV. At Chicken Grammy's house I first viewed the movie that influenced my life more deeply than any other: *The Wizard of Oz*.

I watched this classic film for the first time while snuggled behind Chicken Grammy on a cozy brown velvet sofa in their rambling top-floor family room.

I loved sitting on the couch behind my plump, jolly grandmother, poking my head out from under her arm to see the screen, praying she wouldn't have gas again. Lying behind Chicken Grammy was a dangerous prospect. This is something one doesn't forget.

Then it happened – no, not the gas, thank goodness – my first experience with the dazzling city of emeralds and those brave deeds and magical lands on the other side of the rainbow. In this vibrant, exquisite place, anything could happen, if only you believed. Beyond the eye-popping visual effects, *The Wizard of Oz* touched my soul because for the first time during my young life I was pulled away from constant worry over where Mom was and why she couldn't take care of us, and where Dad was and why he wasn't caring for us. For once I didn't think about not belonging anywhere. This amazing film carried me to a comforting fantasy world where everything was saturated with color, teeming with quirky new friends, and surrounded by enchantment and hope.

I hadn't thought about this feeling place for years, until I awakened to the greeting of my furry piranha.

~ ~ ~ ~

I pry my fingers from Mojo's tenacious grip and gently guide her to the floor. Pulling on my pink fleece pullover, I hurry downstairs with Mojo pouncing behind me, her bushy tail straight in the air as we head for my laptop. No one else is awake, so I bask in the morning silence, broken only by the ticking clock in the kitchen. I need this quiet time to clear my head and tame my racing thoughts. So many emotions swirl through my brain this morning, lost feelings nudging me through the fog.

Mojo climbs onto my lap and paw-presses herself into just the right position, her amber-green eyes surrounded by whiskers, staring up at me with approval.

I begin typing:

> I awakened this morning with a profound sense of destiny. I feel it on every level of my being without question or hesitation. Is this pint-sized angel of a cat warming my heart, inspiring me to believe again?
>
> I feel compelled to write *our* story, a story that has yet to unfold; a story I hope to create within my life. Writing puts events into perspective like a pathway to the truth, bringing

> focus and meaning to my thoughts. I believe voicing my prayers will help bring my dreams into reality. Who better than a mother to manifest a cure for her child?
>
> I see Emma free from the prick of needles, free to enjoy her life unencumbered by worry, free from diabetes. I have no idea how or when, but I'm willing to be patient, because I know somehow this will happen. During insecure moments I feel like Dorothy, searching for a way to get home to the magical place where miracles reside. If only I can find my way to that mystical land where sidewalks sparkle in the sunlight.

I look down at my snuggled kitten, her purr vibrating into my very soul. A wave of peace washes over my tired spirit. Seeing Mojo's perfection, her innocence, makes me believe anything is possible – that I am worthy of my heart's desires, and I *will* find a way to this magical place. I need only to believe.

Chapter 2

Finding Mojo

WILL IS THE FIRST TO COME DOWNSTAIRS. Normally, he crawls into bed with me for a snuggle each morning before starting his day, but he didn't find me drooling peacefully on my pillow this morning.

"Why are you down here, Mommy?" he asks in a sleepy voice, his much-loved baby blanket caressing the sides of his sweet little face.

"This rascal bit my toe," I say, pointing to my lap.

Will's eyes open all the way, and he gently reaches out to pet our newest family member. His gentle touch on Mojo's soft fur reminds me of the times I brought him along on my veterinary ultrasound calls. He's always calm and loving with animals.

I ruffle his silky, platinum blonde hair. "I guess it's time to get ready for school. I'll go wake up Emma."

I hand him our kitten and head upstairs. Emma's usually the last one asleep each night, and therefore the last one up in the morning. I think she finds sleeping a waste of valuable time, but she's a kid and can't stave it off indefinitely – although she tries.

Pastel multicolored hearts glow on the walls of Emma's room. The roller-shade rattles when I pull it open. I pause for a few moments to gaze at Emma's peaceful, sleeping face, her blonde wavy hair flowing along the length of her pillow. Then I scan her chest for signs of breathing, as mothers do the world over. I've always done this, even pre-diabetes. But now I'm prepared at a moment's notice for a crisis. Last night her blood sugars were running high. Her last insulin correction was at 3:00 a.m., so I'm hopeful we're back on track. I'm still amazed how something as simple as a blood sugar value can mess up the rest of our day.

Emma's blood sugar stability is often short lived, which is why I test her during the night, and why I'm often tired in the morning when I should feel rejuvenated.

I run my hand along the length of Emma's arm and then gently rock her back and forth.

"Emma, honey, time to get up. Will has a purring fur ball downstairs who wants to say good morning to you."

Emma awakens slowly, and I stare into those wise, old-soul eyes I fell in love with the day she was born. So much knowledge lies behind those big, blue pools of curiosity. "Would you please ask Will to bring her upstairs for me?" She puts one hand on her face to shield it from the sunlight.

I smile to myself at her request. Even when she was two years old, Emma spoke in long, clear sentences. She skipped right past baby talk and began entrancing grown-ups with her delightful ability to communicate.

~~~~

My children are everything to me. I'm not sure exactly when this happened. At one time I easily combined parenting with my social life: dinner parties, a glass of wine, celebrations, and community events. I was quite active. But now life is *just* about my kids. I don't have the desire or energy for much else. Moreover, I developed an aversion to holidays that involve sweet-toothing our children straight into sickness. Halloween is my least favorite event, what with roaming around in the dark collecting sugary treats that wreak havoc on teeth and immune systems, not to mention blood sugars. I truly don't get it. Obviously, my disdain for Halloween is greater since diabetes entered our lives.
~~~~

I struggle not to become an introverted recluse, which is far from the person I used to be. But my priorities had to change. I can't afford to be tipsy on wine should Emma have a blood sugar problem. I can't afford to feel even more tired than I usually do after a night of socializing. And now that I'm not working, I certainly can't afford new clothes to fit the changes in my body. Gaining weight is a hazardous side effect of relentless interrupted sleep.

~ ~ ~ ~

Will comes upstairs and holds Mojo in front of Emma. He's not ready to hand over the kitten just yet. Emma sits up with an excited smile on her face; I sense the wheels turning in her head as she formulates a plan that will convince Will to cooperate.

"Do you feel 'low' honey?" I ask.

"Nope, I'm good."

I'm grateful Emma can feel her low blood sugars, which is something she could become desensitized to if she had too many. Since she isn't pale or shaky, I decide her morning glucose can wait until breakfast is ready.

I head downstairs to the kitchen, wondering how long Emma will be patient for her turn to hold Mojo. Gazing into the fridge I pull out the ingredients for my newly-discovered health obsession: a kefir, berry, spirulina, Greens Plus shake, brimming with vitamins. Then I whip up our weekday usual: cheese omelets, whole grain toast, and fresh grapefruit. For me, breakfast is the most important meal of the day – and my favorite.

I hear Emma, ever the diplomat, trying to persuade Will. "Would you like to play with my snow globe for a minute while I hold her? I promise to give her back to you." Emma's self-confidence and ability to control her environment are her biggest strengths – attributes of a born leader. She's my creative and engaging *ancient* child.

Will is energetic and compassionate. Born three years after Emma, he felt like an easier baby, although perhaps *I* was more relaxed the second time around. Sleeping was a breeze for Will, except when he'd stay up giggling and baby talking in his crib as though a crowd of invisible fans cheered him on.

One night when I still enjoyed entertaining, several friends and I gathered around the baby monitor in amusement as Will laughed as if being tickled. After an hour of non-stop laughing, I snuck upstairs to peek into his room and see what the heck was going on. I half expected to glimpse, oh I don't know ... maybe an angel tickling him with a feather. When I opened the door, there he was, standing in his crib and smiling at me, completely innocent and apparently alone.

Will always seemed younger than his sister as far as souls go, ready to try anything in his carefree, funny way.

~ ~ ~ ~

I count the carbs in the toast and smoothie, and then write the numbers on the dry erase board on my fridge.

"Time for breakfast!" I call up the stairs.

Emma tests her blood sugar: 5.2 – perfect for us. Normal blood sugars run between 4 to 10 mmol, the Canadian unit of measurement (American would be 72 to 180 mg/dl). Anything below 4mmol is hypoglycemia – low blood sugar – and above 10 mmol is hyperglycemia – high blood sugar. Being in a happy mood can help promote a normal blood sugar. Mojo is excellent for keeping Emma relaxed and content, spreading her good vibes to our entire family.

"When does Dad get home?" Will asks, a bit of egg falling from his lip.

"Friday, by bedtime," I reply. "Only three more sleepies."

Marc's only away a week this time around, which is better than a two-week run. At least the kids will keep busy with school during most of this absence. When I married Marc, I never anticipated I'd spend so much time alone. In fact, I sometimes refer to myself as a single-married woman. My mother-in-law tries to make me feel better by pointing out that Army wives can be alone for months at a time. Somehow, this doesn't comfort me. I didn't marry a man fighting for his country. I married a man who worked regular hours at a desk job in a fiberboard plant with excellent benefits and three weeks paid vacation a year.

However, when companies expand and opportunities for advancement arise, one shouldn't complain about being alone. At least that's what I tell myself.

As Emma and Will finish their breakfasts, I double-check that we provided the right amount of insulin from Emma's pump for her meal. Then I label all the carbs in her lunch. With only minutes to spare until the school bell rings, we hop into my Honda Odyssey and race the six blocks to school, making it just in time.

I return home to my still warm cup of green tea and head back to the laptop I left on the loveseat in the living room. Mojo has managed to climb onto the keyboard and is curled up into a tiny, breathing, ball of fur, enjoying the computer's radiant heat.

"Off the laptop, little one. This isn't the place for a nap."

Sleepy-eyed, she looks up at me, remaining relaxed and floppy as I gently move her to the kitty pillow on the floor. Enticed to write a little more, I drift back to the day I found our ray of sunshine, the day I finally began listening to my instincts once again.

Two Weeks Earlier ~ May 2007

A gentle drizzle tapped against the windshield as I drove home from my spiritual psychology course. I stared at the grey horizon and felt the urge to take a different road. Although I didn't know this area well, the majestic beauty of Lake Nipissing drew me to explore a new route along its shore. This detour would add twenty minutes to my trip, but I was up for a change of scenery, a mini-adventure.

I turned left on Fisher Street, off Highway 11, then right on Main which runs along the water. Everywhere I looked, shimmering green buds sprouted from trees along the road. To my left, glistening water called to me.

Spring is a big deal in northern Ontario. When the snow finally melts I literally feel my soul expand, stretching as if it's been sleeping with the bears all winter long. The misty rain enhanced the rich greens of the awakening trees. My senses heightened, I noticed rays of light piercing the clouds, creating tiny rainbows in the water droplets left behind on my windshield.

I felt calm and focused after spending time with my group of like-minded spiritual seekers. When the road veered away from the lake, I decided to work my way home. Slowing to a near stop I checked the intersection for an exit to the highway when I noticed a sign on my right: Animal Shelter.

I'd always had a pet and I adore animals, but three years earlier Emma tested positive to allergies, forcing us to give away our two Siamese kitties. Will couldn't remember Mitsu and Cleo; he was just a baby. But Emma remembered, and she desperately wanted another cat. In fact, she posted a list on the wall beside her bed in hopes of bringing a new kitten into our lives. A kitten that...

- no one will be allergic to,
- will shed very little,
- will be friendly with everyone,
- will be healthy and loving.

Hating to disappoint her, I researched and found a special breed of hypoallergenic cat—*for fifteen thousand dollars*. If we had that kind of money to throw around, I'd rather sign up for a tummy tuck, or renovate the kitchen.

Even when Emma put out a kitty bowl with food in the corner of our dining room, I still didn't see how her dream could come true. We couldn't risk allergy attacks on top of her diabetes – could we?

But there I was, standing in front of the animal shelter. What harm could it do to look inside? Emma would never know.

I entered the building during happy hour in the cat quarters. Most of the felines were in the common room, frolicking on carpeted tree houses or playing with string balls. I scanned the room, admiring all the different colors and patterns of my favorite creatures, fully expecting to have a bit of fun for a few minutes before getting back in my van and returning home.

Then I noticed the wall of cages with the largest one labeled KITTENS. I couldn't resist opening the latch and diving in. One kitten attracted me over all the others. She had mostly black, long fur with the slightest hint of red-brown tabby stripes. She sat quietly in the corner of the cage away from the others and stared straight at me, as if she knew who I was.

I had to pick her up. As I pulled her close to me, instead of squirming or acting anxious, she stretched up, closed her eyes halfway, and gently kneaded her tiny kitty fingers into my shirt. I looked down at her; she peered up at me through half-open eyes.

I've been waiting for you, she said with a look.

Have you ever known right away when something's meant for you? When it's part of your destiny? For us, this was love at first sight. I knew this kitten and she knew me. I didn't intend to get a pet, not consciously. When I wavered, the fellow on duty assured me we had up to thirty days to return her if anyone in the family showed signs of being allergic.

My brain went into overdrive, rationalizing. Maybe this kitten would be one of those rare, hypoallergenic cats. Better yet, perhaps Emma had outgrown her allergy. I was willing to give it a try.

I held her tiny body in the cradle of my arm, gently smoothing the fur around her ears. Mesmerized by her contented gaze, I relaxed into a blissful state, and her name flashed into my mind: Mojo. She was good energy, like a favorite old song buried deep inside my soul. I felt a glimmer of something that had been missing for too long – something I eagerly wanted to reclaim.

~ ~ ~ ~

Mojo begins to stir. The bubbling of our aquarium lures her toward the swirling, tri-colored angelfish inside. I sip the last of my tea and contemplate why I was drawn to her that day.

I can't take credit for bringing Mojo into our lives. That credit belongs to Emma, who prayed for her to come every night before she fell asleep; Emma, who felt a deep knowing about how important this kitten would be for our family; Emma, who has a knack for doing this sort of thing – creating a need within herself that inevitably fulfills a need of my own.

This train of thought leads me to a dilemma, however: What kind of need could possibly be filled by developing a disease?

Chapter 3

Searching for Courage

A Year and a Half Earlier ~ December 2005

I NOTICED EMMA LOOKING THINNER while we were swimming at our local indoor pool. I shrugged it off as part of a growth spurt, figuring she just needed more calories. Over the next few days I offered her as many of her favorite meals as I could think of: pasta, burgers, home-baked cookies, and muffins. To my delight, she wolfed everything down and asked for more. She'd never been a big eater, so I was excited to see her so voracious. Her drinking also improved, which left me even more curious, because I'd always lorded over her to finish whatever beverage she had on the go. It seemed, finally, she had crossed a new threshold, getting over that awkward, childhood picky eating phase.

The more carbs I shoveled into Emma, the more unusual her condition appeared. She'd eat her entire meal, but cry a half hour later that she was still hungry. This felt a bit annoying, and I wondered if it was a ploy for attention. She couldn't possibly *still* be hungry!

Then Emma's drinking increased exponentially. I'd line up at least four cups of water at bedtime, yet that wasn't enough to get her through the night. I quickly lost my newfound enthusiasm to keep her hydrated. This was beyond the normal health requirements of any seven-year-old.

The morning after Emma had an accident and wet her bed – something she'd never done before, not even while toilet training – I called our doctor. I expected his secretary (whom I'll call Raven) to give me the cold shoulder, as always. I can't explain why, but this woman disliked me from our first hello. I never felt comfortable going in for appointments, and the more I tried to be nice, the more anyone within a square block could sense her irritation.

Raven answered the phone, and I began explaining Emma's situation – something I'd worked on since going to bed the night before. I expressed my concern about Emma's weight loss of six pounds, which, for a little girl who only weighed fifty, was significant. I described how each vertebra in her spine poked out and how her hair was falling out in clumps. The topper was her excessive drinking and bed-wetting.

I heard nothing on the other end of the phone. Just dead air. Total radio silence. No, "Oh, dear, that is concerning. Give me a moment to ask the doctor."

Instead, Raven put me on hold, leaving me wondering if she'd just hung up. How ridiculous for me to feel guilty about bothering this woman at a time when my daughter needed help. *Am I the typical overreacting mother making a big fuss over nothing*? I wondered.

After a few minutes, just when I was about to give up and redial, Raven came back on the line.

"You can bring Emma in after lunch to see the doctor," she said.

"Right. Great! I'll see you then." I hung up, relieved to have accomplished my goal. I mentally prepared myself to face her in a few hours.

I picked up Emma from school and we headed to her appointment. Even though I'm a trained healthcare provider, somehow I'd protected myself from imagining anything serious could be going on. I completely ignored the fact that Emma's symptoms were textbook diabetes; my mind focused on a simple, fixable answer.

Maybe she picked up a parasite on that horrible vacation we had last spring, I told myself.

The visit with our doctor was brief. He wasn't sure if anything was wrong with Emma, but to be prudent, he ordered blood tests that would be drawn the next morning after she fasted all night.

I wish I'd known a simple urine test in his office would have shown ketones and glucose. (Ketones are a toxic byproduct indicative of dissolving fat stores, a result of extreme dieting or starvation.) But *no*, Emma would suffer four more days, because the next morning was Friday, and then we had to get through the weekend before we could see her lab results.

By Sunday I was no longer in denial about my daughter being in serious trouble. I was sleeping with her at night to help her get to the bathroom. Well, if you can call it sleeping. Mostly I lay watching her, waiting for a twitch or moan that might indicate she needed to be awakened for a dash to the toilet.

Emma began complaining of terrible headaches and stomach pains after eating carbohydrate-loaded meals. The sparkle in her eyes dulled. In hindsight, I wish beyond all wishes that I'd thrown my insecurity about my gut feelings aside and taken her to the hospital emergency room that weekend. But I trusted the doctor we had at this time, unaware I could get answers before Monday.

Today, I know my little girl was literally starving to death before my eyes. Her insulin-producing cells were under attack by her immune system, and she could no longer process glucose to fuel her body. The food she ingested couldn't be utilized without insulin. Her blood, now toxic from high blood sugars, forced her kidneys into action to remove the excess glucose through the urine. The more carbs I gave her, the higher her blood sugar soared, which would have been high even without the extra carbs.

I suspect another day or two would have found Emma in a coma from a toxic state known as diabetic ketoacidocis or DKA, which is the most common way parents learn of their child's type 1 diabetes.

On Monday, the doctor's phone lines were busy, so I headed straight to his office. I needed the blood test results, but they still weren't in.

"Then I'd like Emma to see a pediatrician, right away!" I said, standing at the reception window. I could barely keep from shrieking. It's not as if Emma looked like a child on death's door. Thin and pale, yes, but she suffered quietly. My incredible sense of urgency was born of an internal prompting I couldn't properly explain. I'd just spent the last four days watching my daughter waste away, and these people needed to trust my mother's intuition.

"Could I please get a referral to a pediatrician?" I pleaded.

Raven stepped forward. I repeated my request, but I knew she was completely done with me. With no restraint in her expression, she rolled her eyes as if to say, *You're such a hypochondriac; I wish people like you would take a long walk off a steep cliff.*

Now it was official: I was a troublemaker. Having worked in this field for over a decade, I see how easily people get labeled. We healthcare providers remove ourselves, or at least keep hysterical clients at arm's length, in order to stay sane. If we allowed ourselves to feel the pain of every tragic case before us, we'd leap out the nearest twenty-story window. I get it. But her reaction crossed the line for me. If I could have dropped a house on her jet-black curls in that moment, I would have. Two could play at this game.

"I take it you don't have any children," I said, ever so sweetly, knowing she didn't. With one hand on her broomstick, she shot me a spine-chilling glare. I refused to look away. My daughter was sick and I needed answers.

God knows I've been through a lot of stress this past year. Could my judgment be clouded? Have I become unreasonable, a hypochondriac? How does a woman know when she's gone over the edge?

A wave of insecurity squelched my desire to yell at this woman – a visceral gut-wrenching pull at the very core of my being. Then, contrary to my instincts, I bit the inside of my check, hard ... and backed down. I'd have to wait for the test results.

Defeated and feeling sorely misunderstood, I pretended to be patient once again. With a deep breath and a deeper knowing that we shouldn't be waiting for a stupid blood test, I continued to wait.

Emma and I regrouped. She was exhausted and peeing constantly, but the eager student in her wanted to keep things as normal as possible. I let her go to school for a few hours while I anxiously paced the floor at home. Even Emma's teacher expressed concern at how frequently she was running to the bathroom. I assured her we should have answers by the day's end. Finally, by 2:00 p.m., we got the call to come back in. Raven sounded sheepish.

When we arrived at the doctor's office, she immediately escorted us straight to an examination room.

This is unusual. It can't be good.

"Is your husband with you?" my doctor asked.

My husband had an uncanny knack of being out of the country whenever a crisis raged. I braced myself and replied, "No, he's in South Carolina. What are we dealing with?"

Emma sat on my lap, leafing through a book. My doctor looked at me with intense gravity.

As if he were speaking through a tunnel, I heard: "Emma has diabetes. You need to drive her immediately to North Bay. A pediatrician is waiting for you there."

More babbling followed: something about blood work and her diagnosis. All I cared about in this moment was one thing.

"Is there a cure?"

"No," he replied, his face somber. "She'll require multiple injections of insulin every day for the rest of her life."

Emma became stiff in my arms. Until this point she'd been sitting quietly, swinging her legs back and forth and reading, seemingly uninterested in our grown-up concerns.

"Needles!" she squeaked, her eyes probing me for reassurance this wasn't about her. Emma was terrified of needles. Being only seven, she couldn't understand the scope of our conversation, but she *did* know about needles and had endured several last spring before our horrible attempt at a vacation. If there was one thing in the world she hated, it was needles.

I did my best to downplay the news, and focused instead on the fact that she would soon be feeling better. No point in both of us breaking down. I wrapped my arms around my little girl, squeezed her firmly, and gently kissed her forehead, hoping to hide my fear from both Emma and our doctor.

"We'll get you feeling better, sweetie," I said. "We just need to see another doctor in North Bay who can show us what to do."

This all seemed like a bad dream. Even before conceiving Emma, I'd spent every waking moment learning everything I could about how to produce a happy, healthy child. What did I do wrong? How could I take the fear and pain she was about to bear away from her? I'd gladly take it on myself, if only I could.

In stunned silence, we headed home while I tried to process the news. Somehow, in my traumatized state, I was supposed to drive Emma safely to North Bay. My doctor had told us we could be away for a week. I had only minutes to make my arrangements and go.

~ ~ ~ ~

(May I suggest to any doctors who find their patients in a similar situation: Don't ask a distraught, worried mother to drive her sick child almost 200 kilometers in wintry conditions. That's a bad plan. Arrange for them to get to their destination safely, please.)

~ ~ ~ ~

Logistically, the situation felt like a mess. Should I bring Will, who was only four, or break the rules and leave him 24/7 with Astrid, our live-in au pair from Austria who'd only arrived four months earlier? My overprotective nature didn't want to let him out of my sight, but I knew I couldn't keep him occupied in a boring hospital room for an entire week. Thank goodness I had

Astrid. Her concern for Emma equaled mine as she frantically Googled to try and understand the evil we were up against. She helped us collect clothes, games, and books to keep us occupied during our stay, and assured me Will would be in good hands until Marc arrived back home.

With my confused and frightened daughter crying from hunger, thirst, and the need to pee every twenty minutes, I struggled to keep my head on straight and get her to the hospital.

The ride seemed endless as I made up dozens of different arguments to her, explaining why she couldn't have something to eat on the road. Veggies or cheese would have been a suitable snack, as they're carb-free and don't raise blood sugars, but what did I know?

I made several phone calls trying to reach Marc, who was out of cell phone range on a South Carolina construction site. I called my mother-in-law and tried to explain what was happening, while Emma's sobs grew louder and more distressed from the backseat.

It was December 12th and the roads were covered with ice and snow. I searched blindly for the hospital sign, feeling more and more anxious with every cry Emma uttered. I tried desperately to stay calm and collected ... just ten more minutes. I'd even take five, but when I drove up to a red light *too* fast ... *whoosh*. I went straight through the light and into the passenger side of another car! Oh my God, you have got to be kidding me!

This was a perfect time to teach my daughter some eloquent new words.

I pulled my vehicle over to the side, trembling. The other driver and his passenger were approaching me with angry faces. But at least they were walking.

I looked into the backseat at my precious daughter, her eyes wide with fear. Her mom was obviously in no shape for driving. How could I be so careless?

With unusual perception and pity, the men I'd hit grasped my predicament quickly. I definitely could *not* wait around for the police to report our collision. We exchanged numbers. I put my headlight and bumper in the back of the van and off I went. So close, yet so far. Thank goodness the accident wasn't more serious.

Shaken and confused, I pulled into the hospital. True to form, my distress pulled in yet another glitch. I was at the *wrong hospital!* Nobody told me there were *two* in this town. I was so frustrated at this point that I actually began laughing – the kind of maniacal laugh I imagined crazy people emit right before they murder someone. Poor Emma was now worried about *me*, actually forgetting her hunger and thirst for a moment.

By the time I found the right place, the people who were expecting us thought we were a no-show. I tried to act like an intelligent healthcare professional, not a mother on the verge of needing urgent psychological intervention.

Emma's blood sugar was off the charts, literally, so they sent a sample to the lab for a quick check. This meant Emma would have to wait a little longer before she could eat, as they first needed to calculate how much insulin she needed. My brave girl was so hungry and confused. *Didn't we understand how starved she was?*

At last the verdict came in and she could have a huge plate of food, but first she needed to have a needle.

"You'll let me eat if I have that needle?" she forced out through her tears.

"Yes," the pediatrician replied, almost making it sound exciting.

"I'm so hungry, Mommy... I'll take the needle," she whimpered.

My throat swelled and my heart moved up, trying to escape my body. I couldn't cry *too*; I had to be strong for her. I fully expected a larger battle over taking a needle, but she was so tired and hungry at this point that she crumbled like a house of cards in a windstorm. We were both exhausted now and grateful to be in the care of a capable medical team – a team who would show us how to keep Emma alive from this point forward.

~~~~
~~~~

Our first night in the hospital was the most memorable. We shared the room with a teenage girl we later learned was struggling with anorexia. Our bed was nearest the hallway. With the drapes closed around us for privacy, I snuggled with Emma on the bed, holding her in my arms as though she was still my baby. I opened the new scholastic book order she'd received that morning from her teacher and began reading what would become one of her favorite childhood books: *Skippyjon Jones* – a story about a Siamese cat with ears too big for his head. This delightful story made us laugh at a time when nothing else seemed funny.

A nurse came in several times during the night to check Emma's blood sugar. She told us Emma needed checks even while sleeping because it was possible for her to have a low blood sugar level and go into insulin shock without waking. Emma and I looked at each other with shock in our eyes. That moment was the end of Emma feeling safe to fall asleep alone and the end of me sleeping through a full night.

We spent the rest of the week in the hospital learning the ins and outs of living with a pancreas that could no longer do its job. (A pancreas, by the way, is a lumpy, elongated gland located below the curve of the duodenum, off the stomach – in the centre of the abdomen. It secretes pancreatic digestive enzymes and insulin.) I was happy to acquire the bed next to Emma when our roommate left the day after we arrived. Sleep deprivation had already begun to set in.

We learned how type 1 diabetes (also called juvenile diabetes, although adults can also get T1) is a completely different entity than type 2 diabetes. Type 1 is an autoimmune disease that destroys insulin-producing cells. Before the invention of insulin, life expectancy with type 1 diabetes was only a matter of weeks, or perhaps months if you underwent a starvation diet. Type 2 occurs when the body's cells are insulin resistant or the pancreas cannot keep up with demands, either through genetics, obesity, or old age.

Type 2 is potentially reversible with aggressive diet and exercise. Type 1 is incurable.

I researched the complications that can occur with poor control of diabetes: eye, nerve, heart, and kidney damage; a shorter life expectancy; and life threatening high or low blood sugars.

I learned how to count carbs, calculate insulin, pin Emma down, and give her a needle at the same time. I began crafting diligent logs on my laptop in order to track trends in her eating and insulin needs. We saw nutritionists and psychologists, as well as family services, hoping for financial assistance (which we didn't qualify for because of Marc's income).

Even though my career training as a medical imaging technologist helped me understand the pathology and physiology of this disease, I still felt overwhelmed by the amount of information thrown at me. I can't imagine for one minute how a non-medically trained person could begin to absorb this much detail in such a short time.

Emma soon felt better once the right doses of insulin were established, and she eagerly ate any food the hospital staff offered. Now that her body was able to absorb glucose, she had a lot of ground to make up.

Within a couple of days, Emma's strength returned and the realities of her new existence came into focus. She would need to be jabbed with needles for painful insulin injections at least four times a day, plus a minimum of eight pokes to the ends of her tender little fingers for glucose checks. We'd have to count the amount of carbs in everything she ate, taking into account the delicate balance of food and exercise, combined with severe fluctuations caused by stress, illness, and growth spurts.

Giving needles would become very unpleasant, as she would resist and resent them more and more with each one. Needles are still the most difficult part of this disease for Emma to accept, even as I write these words.

~ ~ ~ ~

On our final night in hospital, I looked out the window into the night while Emma slept. Fresh snow fell on the cars in the parking lot below, and neighboring houses sparkled with Christmas lights and decorations. I pictured families snug and warm in their cozy homes, preparing for Santa, family gatherings, and turkey feasts.

The night was so quiet. Acutely aware of everything around me, I could hear myself breathe. *What would be next for us?* The things I considered important only days ago no longer mattered. I knew, without a second thought, that I would not be able to travel and run my veterinary ultrasound business, a business I'd developed on my own and was gratified by each day.

I had one week to make Christmas normal at a time when nothing felt normal. I needed to teach Marc all that I'd learned, and somehow comfort Will while Emma cried and screamed during her injections. I knew Astrid wouldn't be able to stay on with the loss of my income. I would have to find a way to do all these things on my own, because now, more than ever, Marc's job was crucial. He had to know I could handle this; I had to be strong. I would need to keep Emma's blood sugars within the proper ranges to avoid life-threatening highs and lows. Everything was about to change.

I turned and looked at Emma's beautiful little face. She seemed so young and fragile, reminding me of earlier times when she was younger, and yet still so wise – back when we first moved to the big, beautiful house in our serene town. Emma was only three, sitting contently on my left hip while I scurried about, trying to find a missing box with important baby items for Will. I couldn't find it anywhere. Emma enjoyed riding on my hip as I searched the many levels of our new home.

Feeding Emma's love for words, I began verbalizing my concerns for the lost box aloud. "How *awful*," I said. "It would be a real *disaster* if it was lost ... *devastating* ... *tragic* ... *CATASTROPHIC,* even!" I exaggerated each word, knowing Emma absorbed every syllable.

She looked at me with her big, serious blue eyes and marveled at all the huge words I'd uttered, soaking them in for later use on unsuspecting grownups. Then she smiled as the new input was fully processed.

With prideful understanding, she declared, "Yeah, that's right. The *CATS* did it."

We still had Mitsu and Cleo at this time, and boy, did we ever blame those cats for every chewed-up electrical cord, missing hair elastic, mangled plant, or those revolting puddles of coughed-up hairballs that always landed on our beautiful carpet.

If only those cats were around to blame for this one.

Missing a few possessions was one thing. Missing critical cells in your body is another situation entirely. I longed to turn the clock back to that younger Emma; to rewind life, sort out what went wrong within her body, and stop it from happening. I couldn't justify why Emma should be forced to live the rest of her life like this. I felt the need to take as much of the burden from her as I possibly could. Life can be difficult enough without the daily threat and balancing act of critical blood sugar levels. How would she cope with all these changes? She would have to search for courage; we would *both* need courage to get through this.

A small part of my awareness began connecting the dots. This wasn't the only catastrophe for the year. It had definitely been the worst year of my life. *I must have been missing something – a message from the universe that wasn't sinking in.*

I sat there in the stillness of the night, listening to the whispers of nurses down the hallway. Before she was diagnosed I had ideas of how life *should* be. What people thought of me was always important and I often pushed myself hard, ignoring the needs of my body.

I couldn't ignore the needs of Emma's body. I couldn't ignore the universal sledgehammer repeatedly hitting me over the head this past year. I would need to get back in the driver's seat of my life – not just for me, but for my family.

First, I had a new job to master, as I'd officially become *Emma's pancreas*. I like to think that as far as body organs go, I'm more attractive than the average pancreas. But, I'm definitely a pancreas.

Chapter 4

Our Toto

Back to 2007 ~ October

I CAN BE AWAKENED FROM even the deepest sleep at a moment's notice – a handy skill for a parent. Many times I've opened my eyes to see my son standing by my bed, blanket in hand, staring at me as he tries to assess whether or not he should climb in. The first few times this occurred I found it oddly creepy having someone – even my own flesh and blood – a breath away, observing me silently in the dark. But I was used to it now. Still creepy, but used to it.

Tonight, half dreaming and half alert for anything out of the ordinary, I feel I'm being watched again. Since I've taken over the role of Emma's pancreas, nighttime is an on-duty shift that calls for constant vigilance. Marc's job – the income upon which we now rely – requires him to be alert during the day. That means I'm the one who adjusts to interrupted sleep throughout each night, even when Marc is actually home.

The feeling of being watched persists, so I put my dream on hold and open my eyes to investigate. Instead of my usual blond haired, blue-eyed night stalker, I discover my observer on the bed, inches from my face.

Mojo is almost invisible in the dark bedroom, her black fur blending into the night. If I hadn't trained myself to expect nocturnal visitors, she might have gained a license to fly tonight, because her whiskers feel like spider legs crawling up my cheek. I reach out to wipe the trail of moisture along my ear, resisting the urge to giggle. *Her nose is so cool and wet. I've never noticed that.*

"What are you doing here, Mojo?"

Mojo doesn't normally come into my bed at night. If she isn't patrolling for mice in the kitchen, she's curled up beside the human who manifested her: Emma. I reach out to pet her, but she jumps to the floor, trots to the doorway, and looks back at me. She wants me to follow; there's no mistaking the message. She's speaking to me with her eyes.

I glance at the clock: 2:00 a.m. I don't normally get up for another hour to check Emma's blood sugar. Nevertheless, I'm awake now, so I may as well. Mojo waits while I visit the bathroom, barely containing her impatience.

"What? Can't a girl go to the washroom?"

I follow Mojo into Emma's room and she jumps onto the bed, watching my every move. *This is new. I've never seen her so curious about my nightly routine.* I put a fresh, sharp lancet into the holder and pull back the pin, then take a new test strip out and place it into the meter. Next, a wet tissue to clean one of Emma's delicate little fingers. It always amazes me how soundly she sleeps at night. Even if a fire alarm rang she wouldn't stir. When I jab the sharp lancet into the end of her finger to squeeze out a drop of blood, she doesn't flinch. I suppose this is a good thing.

The glucose strip draws up the blood that collects on the tip of her finger. I watch the meter as it counts down to read out her blood sugar: 2.5.

I blink in surprise. A reading of 2.5 is much too low. Because Emma is such a sound sleeper, she wouldn't recognize the signs of hypoglycemia: dizziness, hunger, and shaking hands. She could slip into a seizure, unconsciousness, and even death.

I reach over to pet my little helper. "Nice catch, Mojo. Is this why you woke me?"

Mojo gazes at my face while I praise her noble efforts to help me do my job. Her eyes close partway in approval. Then, with a quiet meow, she jumps off the bed and heads over to the window ledge.

Emma's blood glucose bottoms out at least one night a week. This never seems to correspond to a specific activity or meal; nothing I can track on a grid. It's more like a cyclic rhythm of her body. High blood sugars are more common for Emma, requiring me to check her every hour until I get the level under control. However, low blood sugars usually take less than a half-hour to bring back up. Usually.

I gently awaken Emma long enough to slurp down an oversized juice box, munch on some cheese, and eat a handful of gluten-free pretzels. Emma doesn't have an issue with gluten (AKA celiac disease) as many T1's do; we just like those pretzels. She closes her eyes even before she lays her head back onto the pillow. I turn the basal rate on her insulin pump down twenty percent for the rest of the night and will wait for fifteen minutes before checking her blood sugar again.

I move over to the window and sit down next to Mojo, who's gazing out into the night. There's no point going back to bed, so I pet her long, soft fur and marvel at the bright autumn sky. The moon is full tonight, and the energy it sends makes me feel stronger somehow. I breathe in its power through my skin and contemplate how nice it is to have a helper, a furry friend to share my night shift, like my very own Toto.

I turn to look at Emma again. She looks so peaceful as she sleeps, like an angel. A barrage of questions flood into my mind.

Why *do* children get diseases? I can understand how adults build up to disease, based on factors such as endless stress, poor lifestyle choices, and perhaps years of suppressed emotions. But what about newborns, or well-nurtured, happy children?

As a mother, I feel responsible for the health and welfare of my children. I know I'm not the only one who thinks this way. Why did my daughter's body stop working properly? Could it be something in our environment or food? Is it related to immunizations? I find it hard to believe this illness is a random event. We have no known genetic history of diabetes on either side of our family. So, what went wrong?

The full moon, so bright I can almost see distinct valleys and craters, draws me back to the sky. Thousands of glittering stars wink at me, their radiance hinting of universal mysteries. During these quiet moments I ponder the new concepts I've learned since taking my spiritual psychology course. As a medical imaging technologist I was trained to sleuth out the cause of illness. I'm inclined to explore all possible angles, including the spiritual side to this problem.

My psychology course conveyed that we actually choose our lives while we're in spirit form, before coming to earth. During that period we make contracts with those who are closest to us – contracts to help fulfill our life purposes.

With that theory in mind, I put aside the *how* part of the equation for a moment and consider the *why* – that Emma may have agreed on a spiritual level to take on this burden for some greater benefit, and we, her family, consented.

I find this idea difficult to swallow. If some sort of pre-negotiated pact between us exists, can I change it now? If we do plan our own experiences in life, then why would we plan *this* experience? How can we learn our lesson quickly and move on to better things?

Mojo's purring pulls me back to the room. I check Emma's blood sugar again: 3.8. Sheesh. I won't go back to bed until I see a 7 on the meter, so I head downstairs for another round of snacks. *Do I have any bran muffins left? Did Emma get extra exercise at school today? Maybe her pancreas is firing back up tonight.*

I rack my brain for clues about why Emma's blood sugar is still low, while I pour more juice past her sweet, sleepy lips.

After feeding Emma again, I return to the window with Mojo, who's entranced by every moonlit shadow in the trees below, trees alive with the makings of feline fantasies and perhaps the answers to the mysteries of the Great Beyond.

Life seems much simpler in the quiet of the night. No racing around to every extracurricular activity known to man in hopes of developing my offspring's budding talents. No buzzing phones. No expectations whatsoever, other than safe blood sugars and sleep. During the day I'm lost in a sea of details, forgetting the juiciness of the moment. Each minute is consumed by planning what comes next. Everything seems to be about accomplishing a future goal, like being on that proverbial hamster wheel and never arriving.

Before this moment, in my busy adult life, I didn't truly feel what it meant to be *in the moment*, although it's something my children accomplish all the time without even trying. Tonight, I have Mojo helping me. I return to Emma's bedside and take another blood sugar: the reading is 7.9, finally. I crawl back into my cold, empty bed, hopeful to get back to sleep.

6:30 A.M.

I barely close my eyes before the alarm clock beeps at me, a reminder that sleep is not written into the contract of a dedicated surrogate pancreas. I consider letting the whole house stay in bed – a fantasy that crosses my mind *every* morning. I peel my body off the sheets and head to the bathroom for a warm shower, hoping to open my eyes a little wider.

I drop my well-worn pajama bottoms to the floor, slide the shirt over my head, and glimpse myself in the large bathroom mirror surrounded by cedar walls and rich blue ceramic counters. Somehow, I look different this morning. When I was younger I took my body for granted – a thin, blue-eyed blonde with little appreciation for my great genes.

While waiting for the water to heat I stand near the mirror, trying not to look closely at my reflection. I'm too tired to deal with my flaws right now, so I gaze at the top of the mirror where I taped two pictures. On the left is a picture of a golden Buddha that says; *All that we are is a result of what we have thought.*

What an incredible responsibility this spiritual idea suggests. For how many years did I look in the mirror during moments like this, at my fit, young body and find fault with it? What kind of results come from such thoughts?

Until the past year I'd never been serious about spirituality. My interest in the meaning of life began to flicker during my late teens when I read books by Shirley Maclaine and others about Buddhism. I was mostly intrigued by the concepts then; no life-transforming moments occurred. The traditions of church and Godly worship were lost on me. Being inside a church made me uncomfortable. I felt it didn't matter what someone worshiped or prayed to: Allah, Buddha, God, St. Teresa, Archangel Michael, or Elvis. To me, it was a different hat on the head of the same entity. I believed the Creator wore diverse caps to appease multiple cultures and lifestyles here on earth.

So now, here I am, reading a Buddhist saying on my mirror. To the right is a picture of a far-off galaxy with words from Winston Churchill: *You create your own universe as you go along.*

Well, that's probably another way of phrasing Buddha's thought, but it feels more optimistic to me, and more scientific. At one time during my life I did create my own universe as I went along, completely unaware of my true power. This was when I met the two most significant people in my life.

I test the water; it's finally ready, so I tear myself away from the mirror and step under the warm, cascading stream. I pick up Marc's razor, which I'd knocked off the shelf again. I think I do this deliberately each day, perhaps to remind myself I do have a partner in life; a man to keep my bed warm at night when he's not away for his job; a fellow parent to help glue together the pieces of my world when I feel too tired to cope with our new existence.

Marc was one of the significant people who came into my life during my younger high-spirited, sheer-determination-to-do-better years. In those days I rarely had trouble interacting with the opposite sex. What you saw was what you got with no confusing subplots to figure out. I had my first boyfriend as early as grade one, holding hands at recess and sharing our lunch desserts. I found boys easier to relate to than girls, because I could count on them to treat me with kindness and affection. Girls were less predictable and difficult for me to trust.

The day I met the most important boy in my life I felt immediately drawn to him. I was sixteen and on a date at a Christmas party when I first heard Marc's voice. I was compelled to turn my head almost magnetically toward the sound. There he stood, in an adjacent room with *his* date. I walked through the crowd toward him, searching for someone I had never met. Our eyes locked. His voice felt like gravity; his mischievous blue eyes, curly blond hair, and athletic build hijacked my mind. I'm not exaggerating when I say that within ten minutes, we ditched our dates and headed into the night like a couple of fugitives on the run.

This was perhaps the strongest intuitive moment of my life. It felt so natural to be with Marc – almost necessary. The simple touch of his hand sent a surge of fire through my heart. Even at such a young age, somehow I knew we were meant to make an important journey together — a journey that now keeps him away from our family far too often for my liking.

I suppose my life would be easier if I had more female friends to rely on for support while Marc's away, but relationships with women have always been a challenge for me, especially in my younger years. I suspect, deep down, I didn't trust women because they could break my heart more easily than any man. This left me feeling guarded and wary toward female friendships. However, that didn't include Karen, the second significant person in my glory days. Karen managed to move past all my protective filters and find her way into my heart.

We met during our senior year of high school. She was beautiful, funny, and genuine. I didn't need to read between the lines with Karen; we each wore our hearts on our sleeves and trusted one another completely. When I came up with the crazy idea to travel out west once we graduated, she said, "When do we leave?" We packed our gear and headed out on a train, two fearless, confident young women ready to take on the world.

We talked about our dreams of the future – what careers we wanted, what our husbands would be like, where we'd travel, how many kids we hoped for, everything.

We grew into women, chose our husbands and got hitched, which placed us eight hundred kilometers apart. We each threw all our energy into being wives and mothers, and we understood this part of our lives didn't leave much room for a long distance friendship. Without hurt feelings or sentiment, we lost touch. I truly missed having Karen in my life, but perhaps that wasn't in our spiritual contract with each other.

Creating your own universe as you go along. I now believe that's what Karen and I did, because I accomplished everything we fantasized about. I married the man of my dreams, achieved a rewarding career doing ultrasound, traveled to New Zealand (the one place I had always wanted to go), and was blessed with two fantastic children. I was practically invincible ... before everything changed.

~ ~ ~ ~

I turn off the water and leave the steamy shower for my mirrored bathroom. Here I am again—a wet, exhausted, nearly forty-year-old woman. When did that happen? I pause for a moment, then finally give in and look closer. Turning to my right, then to my left. Hmm. Definitely more curvy, but is that so bad?

I dry myself, then pull on my favorite black shirt and faded jeans. Mojo passes by my feet, rubbing the length of her body along my shin.

"Good morning to you too." I say. A new sense of discovery flows into my heart as I remember her heroics last night. Suddenly I don't feel so alone.

"Maybe looking closer into my life isn't such a bad thing, Mojo. It might help me sort out how, and when, I got so far off track."

She stares up at me with those clear, innocent green eyes, and I have a feeling she understands every word.

And now the hard part begins...

Chapter 5

The Storm

Going Back Again ~ One Year Before Diabetes ~ December 2004

NORMALLY, THE WHOLE FAMILY would come to our house during the holidays. The cozy fireplace, hardwood floors, and spacious rooms that flow into one another made our home a perfect gathering spot. This year Christmas would be quieter than usual. Marc's two brothers Bill and Jamie were in Thailand for Bill's wedding to his beautiful Thai fiancée, June, in her family's home city of Bangkok. That left Marc's parents and aunt as our only holiday guests.

My adventuresome spirit longed to be with the other half of the Colvins for the Buddhist wedding ceremony on the opposite side of the world, but we weren't able to share this adventure. Our children were young, three and six, and Marc's dad suffered a stroke the year before Emma was born, so we stayed to hold the fort at home and share the Thai journey via phone calls.

Jamie, Marc's younger brother, called on Christmas Eve to describe the side trip he and *his* fiancée, Adrienne, took to Phuket Island, regaling us with tales of the not-to-be-believed snorkeling, glorious tropical landscape, warm Thai hospitality, and savory food. This sounded intoxicating, entirely opposite the traditional wintery Christmas we were having in Canada.

A fresh layer of snow blanketed the landscape in our snug little town. Emma and Will burst with the anticipation of Santa squeezing his cookie-bloated tummy down our chimney. We felt safe and sound at home in our protective bubble of happiness. Christmas came and went as we relaxed into the holiday season.

Then someone turned on CNN.

Negative stories are no fun; I rarely listen to the news or read newspapers, figuring the truly important stuff will reach me. My news junkie in-laws worry about my lack of interest in the headlines and constantly send clipped articles in the mail, desperate to keep me informed.

After heating our holiday leftovers, I sat down to relax and read the instructions on some of Emma and Will's new toys ... and watch CNN with the family.

Early reports were coming in about an earthquake and possible tidal wave hitting the Island of Phuket.

"Did he just say Phuket?" I asked.

Marc reached for the remote and turned up the volume. We fixed our eyes on the screen, searching for more information.

We were fairly certain Jamie and Adrienne had already left the island, so we decided to wait for them to call and reassure us all was well.

The day came and went, but no call...

We remained glued to the television. The devastation was beyond anything imaginable. The TV echoed throughout the house late into the evening, well after Emma and Will were asleep, only to be turned back on again when Marc's parents arose with the sun. Stories and images of people who'd been swept out to sea flashed across the screen, mostly helpless children who couldn't save themselves. I was sick inside, unable to stand the graphic footage. I wanted to turn my head, but I was obsessed with searching for any indication our family was safe.

On the second day we worked our way through the list of phone numbers we had for the boys, but no luck getting through.

By day three, the thrill of Santa was long gone and our mealtime conversations were muted by somber concerns. Why couldn't we reach anyone? Surely their cell phones still worked. I scrambled to figure out how to call an embassy.

I tried with all my might to tell myself everything was fine. In my mind they were in Bangkok, unharmed. Then terrifying news images would take control of my thoughts, like kidnappers with rifles mangling the fragile images I worked so hard to create. All I could see were millions of people struggling with the reality of dead or missing relatives, destroyed homes, and shattered lives. Thousands of corpses, many hanging in trees or washed up on beaches, rotted in the tropical heat. With no food or clean water, the risk of famine and epidemic disease was high. This could double the death toll to something like 300,000.

The news coverage did an excellent job of horrifying the entire world. Being informed is obviously important, but did we need to know about babies dangling from wire fences? The picture that most plagued my mind came from an individual survival tale, the story of an Australian mother who had to choose which of her two young sons to release while a torrent of water crushed down upon them. All three would perish if she didn't free one of her hands to hang onto something. With the angry, hard rush of ocean thundering in, she had mere moments to make her decision.

The mother chose to let go of her slightly older son, in hopes he might be strong enough to swim. She watched in anguish as the ocean swept him away from her. I pictured myself trying to hold onto the most important things in my life – my children – and felt her torture. I'd rather die than have to choose which child not to protect.

The boy she let go of miraculously survived and was reunited with his mom within a couple of days. In subsequent TV interviews I could see the fear lingering in his eyes. Yes, he survived, but what about the rest of his life? What about the memory of his mother letting him go? I had no idea why this affected me so much, but it was truly more than I could take, pulling at something so deep within me that I wept at each sight of his confused little face.

Finally, the phone rang. Our family was safe at the airport in California, ready to board their connection for home. They'd been in Bangkok during the tsunami, vaguely aware of an earthquake, but without access to the news they had no clue of our concerns and were oblivious to the devastation they escaped.

If I'd known then how important *my thoughts* were, I probably wouldn't be writing this book now. Unfortunately, I didn't, and this is where the "feeling helpless" part of my ride began. Watching the nightmarish images on TV pulled at feelings within me, so strong and long buried, that it triggered my own *emotional* tidal wave: a wave filled with fear and loss of control – leaving children in its wake.

Chapter 6

If I Didn't Have a Heart

February 2005

ONCE MARC'S BROTHERS RETURNED home in one piece, we resumed our normal, comfortable routine. But my thoughts were anything but comforting. The drama of Christmas break became a virus burrowing into the fabric of my consciousness, and I shared the story with anyone who'd listen. I felt as if an old familiar frequency had resurfaced from deep within my cells – slowly, stealthily, sneaking up on me like a predator in the dark.

It didn't take long for me to find the vibration again. Debbie, the sister of my oldest, dearest friend, Karen, phoned me out-of-the-blue. A jolt of excitement rushed through me as I replayed the message, eagerly scribbling down the number to return her call. I'd hated that Karen and I lost touch, and I often thought about tracking her down. Somehow, five or even ten years can pass without noticing.

Debbie's voice was strained; she wasted no time on small talk. She stuttered while searching for words to tell me why she'd spent two days looking for my number.

"I'm sorry to have to phone you with this news Julie, but it's Karen... She's not well. She has breast cancer, and despite a mastectomy and chemo, it's spread quickly. The doctors have only given her weeks to live."

I was silent for a moment, replaying her words. Karen has three children – two boys and a girl. She's a beam of sunshine. There must be a mistake.

I knew there wasn't. My thoughts tumbled. If only I'd stayed in touch. Where is she? Is there time to see her?

"I'm so sorry, Debbie. Is there anything I can do?" I whispered.

She explained that she and Karen were attending the final competition of Karen's synchronized skating team the following weekend. This would be a weekend for them to get away, just the two of them. They'd booked a beautiful hotel and spa to stay in following the event.

"Would you like to join us?"

"Absolutely!" I said, without a second thought.

Fortunately, Marc was home and could stay with Emma and Will. I quickly packed a bag for the weekend and tore myself from my parental responsibilities, the first time away from my family.

The drive went quickly as memories of our teenage years came rushing back. Our grade twelve camping trip to Algonquin Park, which lasted a week longer than planned because of an invitation to stay from the handsome outpost ranger (he looked remarkably like Tom Cruise). Our train adventure to Banff, Alberta after graduating high school – the duration of our stay regretfully cut short this time (another boy involved with changing these plans). My visits to Karen's family farm and the exhilaration of pulling on the hooves of a new calf to free it from its laboring mother. And, there was Karen's uncanny ability to always go the wrong way when traveling. Her bad sense of direction was so reliable that I would deliberately wait for Karen to decide which route to take, then confidently press on in the opposite direction.

Memories came flooding back to me like the spring thaw on a vibrant river, but excited as I was to see my best friend again, I also felt nervous. *Had time changed things? Would it still be easy to talk to her? How should I act around a friend who's dying? Should I mention her cancer or keep it light? Cancer might be the last thing she'd want to talk about. Maybe I should just look at this as a visit with my dearest friend.* I felt pretty sure I could manage that.

The drive was smooth. I squinted through the sun's reflection off the white frozen landscape and arrived on schedule. Debbie planned to sneak me onto the Synchro team bus, a place where Karen would never expect to bump into an old friend.

The clouds seemed to roll in just as I approached the parking lot full of buses and slush. A grey dampness filled the air. With trepidation, I looked at the stairs leading into her noisy, estrogen-filled bus. *Can I do this? I haven't seen Karen for so long; will she even want to see me?*

The warm air of the bus interior blew back my hair and forced me to squint for a moment. I scanned through the glittery maze, searching for the best friend I'd ever known, one of the few women in my life I'd entrusted with a piece of my heart. There she was, standing in the aisle, facing away from me. Her long, curly brown hair was pulled up like the rest of the women, even though she wouldn't be skating today. I was always amazed by how quickly her hair grew.

Anxious to call out her name and see her beautiful face, I pushed past my fear, took a deep breath, and called to her.

"Hey Karen, fancy meeting you here!"

Karen spun around. I must have looked like a ghost standing there – the last person she expected to see. Her liquid-brown, puppy dog eyes, searched for the voice she hadn't heard in years. I could see the pause in her expression as she took a moment to process how I'd gotten there, and then looked over my shoulder at her sister. The smile came, spreading from ear to ear. Her eyes softened as she walked toward me with her arms outstretched. "J-U-L-I-E!"

With that smile I saw the beautiful, bubbly, and genuine girl with whom I'd shared a crucial part of my life. I saw someone else there, too. For a brief second before the grin, I caught a glimpse of a woman struggling to hang onto her spark. Sadness and joy coursed through me at the same time, which can only bring one possible outcome ... Tears!

Our reunion was brief, because Karen and the rest of the team needed to head for the rink and prepare for their competitions. Debbie and I found our way to the arena and caught up on all the gossip:

"Did you hear David finally got married?"

"No, you're kidding! When?"

"You know about Sandra, right? She had six kids!"

"Really! Is she still gorgeous?"

We relaxed into our seats to enjoy the show – and what a show. I'd never seen synchronized skating before; it was so fast and perfectly timed. The routines seemed dangerous to me, but Debbie said the fun outweighed the minimal risk. Fourteen grown women, many of them mothers, wove in and out of complex formations, going at high speed. One wrong turn or trip might lead to a pile-up of glitter and sequins. Who would make lunches on Monday?

The point today wasn't to skate or gossip, but to escape into more peaceful, neutral ground – a necessity for two sisters consumed with the painful reality of planning for death. This weekend would not include funeral details or conversations on last wishes. No. This was about the good old days, the silly things we'd done together, and the fun times we could still have – at least for today. This was a break from reality.

Driving to the hotel that night, Karen joined me in my van and we caught up on our missing years. Our talk was effortless, as if no time had passed. The next day came all too quickly and saw us checking into our elegant spa, a first for me.

Karen and I got pedicures, then I had a fancy body-wrap and a detox thing with oils, hot steamy towels, and an abdominal massage. I've lived most of my adult life with a sensitive internal ecosystem triggered by the wrong foods, stress, or lack of sleep, but didn't think the massage would upset things. Unfortunately, my body couldn't ignore the turmoil I was feeling about Karen's situation. My mind can create whatever shields it needs to protect itself, but the rest of me cannot suppress my emotions.

So, by the time I was back with Karen and Debbie to enjoy the snowy outdoor hot tub, Karen was quick to shout in front of perfect strangers,

"Hey Julie ... how's the diarrhea?"

I laughed so hard I almost did have an accident, in the tub. Not disease, or pain or even a date with death could change the Karen I'd always known – the pure, mischievous soul who was always filled with light and laughter.

When it was time to leave I didn't know how to say goodbye. *What should I say?* "Have a good death; see you on the other side." The mind just can't go there. It protects itself and spins a story about how things will be okay. Somehow, you'll be together again. Maybe the doctors were wrong. Maybe she could recover. I knew this wasn't true, but I couldn't bear thinking of this world without her in it.

I drove home through a blur of tears, trying to reason with myself that death is a part of life, not a "bad" thing. From what I'd read, Buddhist monks spend their whole lives preparing for this moment, the instant they believe we return to source energy and become free of our limiting flesh, ready for a new and improved human life.

It *will* be okay, won't it? She must have accomplished her purpose for this lifetime. But what about the people left behind who would miss her? *What about her children?*

~ ~ ~ ~

I tried to keep in touch with Karen, but she became too frail to reply. Several weeks passed and the phone rang. It was Debbie.

"Karen's slipping away. Do you want to come one last time?"

The hospital was a nine-hour drive, and this time Marc was out of the country.

I absolutely wanted to come, but I would have to wait for Marc to get back, which would likely be too late.

"Please let her know I love her. If Marc can get home, I'll come."

Two days passed and Marc hadn't made it home yet. The phone rang again.

"I don't know why she's holding on, Julie; we can't figure it out. The entire family is here and they say it should be any hour, but then another day passes. One of the nurses asked if she could be waiting for someone. All we can think of is that it's you. We mentioned to her that you would try to come."

My heart fell, breaking into hundreds of tiny, ragged, pieces. I had to get there somehow. I couldn't let her down this way. *Please, God, if you're there ... help me get to Karen!* I've never been one to try prayer, but desperate times call for desperate measures.

"I'll call you right back," I told Debbie, and began pacing and praying even harder for a way to get to Karen. Just as I was about to scream out in frustration, Marc called:

"I found a flight and can be home by bedtime."

Relief surged through me as I obtained the help of my new friend Lois, who filled in the gap of the missing babysitting hours. I packed a small bag and headed off in my van.

~ ~ ~ ~

During the long drive I kept hearing Karen's teenage voice in my head. It was Karen's birthday and I didn't have any money to buy her a present.

"Today's my birthday," she said, with the sad face and voice of Eeyore from *Winnie the Pooh*. We were both broke and she was feeling rightfully sorry for herself. I borrowed enough money to splurge on a chocolate-covered donut and put a candle in it. Her smile was so big. She cut her gift in half and we shared it.

"Today was a great birthday," she said. "The best one ever!"

I kept hearing her voice in my thoughts, "Today's my birthday." Slow and melodically, but today wasn't actually her birthday. *Why am I thinking about this*?

After the ninth hour, it was late at night. I was driving to a place I'd never been to, yet my van seemed to be on autopilot. As I drew closer to the hospital I tried to call Karen's room. No answer.

That's strange; I know they're all with her.

I had no directions to the hospital, and yet I drove straight into the correct parking lot, where two people came out and guided me directly to Karen's room.

I saw Debbie first, her eyes swollen, her nose red.

"She's gone, Julie. Just a few minutes ago."

Karen's whole family sat in the room – her parents, husband, three beautiful children, sister, current best friend (also named Julie), and now me, her oldest, best friend.

All eyes were on me as I entered; her children looked confused, not knowing who I was. Her parents warmly invited me to come in. They hadn't changed a day since I last saw them. Debbie brought me to Karen's side and encouraged me to say goodbye. I looked at the girl who was the brightest ray of sunshine I had ever known – the only female in my life who hadn't somehow broken my heart. All I could see now was an empty shell that used to be Karen. She was no longer the person I'd known, but rather a suitcase she'd traveled in, her light now gone.

I gently picked up her hand and leaned in slowly toward her ear. "Today's your birthday," I whispered. "I love you."

In the silence of the room, I knew her spirit was close. I was sure she helped guide me to her bedside that night. I could see her, not as she was on that bed, but the Karen I'd always known. I saw her in my mind, smiling, free from pain, and full of love for everyone who'd helped her cross over.

I don't believe Karen needed me to be present that night for her to make the transition. I think she wanted me there for Debbie, who lived two hours away – to get her sister safely home to her own young family, a husband and three little girls. Debbie needed to touch neutral ground again, to process her new reality. I was able to do that for Debbie and for Karen.

Several tragic, premature deaths of friends had been scattered throughout my life, but none touched me like this one. None made my heart ache with so much pain that I could feel it struggling to protect itself. If only I didn't have a heart, then it couldn't be broken like this. I felt as if a piece of me died that day.

Again, I felt a sense of having no control over life or death. The sheer devastation of Karen's beautiful children left without a mother triggered more fearful emotions, just like the tsunami.

Maybe I can't protect my family from harm's way. Maybe no one is truly safe!

Chapter 7

If I only had a Brain

May 2005

I GET NERVOUS WRITING ABOUT painful or negative things. I no longer wish to relive those times or risk getting caught up in their downer frequencies. But you wouldn't have guessed it while I was going through these problems – no way. Back then, our "you're not going to believe this" hardships were all I could think or talk about.

"How are you today?" someone would ask me at the grocery counter.

"Oh, not bad, except we almost lost half our family in that horrible tsunami, and then my most treasured friend passed away!" On I'd drone, blah-blah-blah, telling my sad story to anyone who'd listen, until they either passed out or ran away.

Wouldn't you know – on the heels of Karen's death, my favorite granduncle passed away at a respectable age of ninety-two. I was chosen to write George's eulogy and speak at his funeral. Once again Marc was away, so I dealt with another death on my own, the final goodbye to a treasured mentor and friend. When pregnant with Emma I had lived with Uncle George for several months while taking a full-time echocardiography course in Toronto. I would drive home to Marc on the weekends, but diligently studied and grew rounder during weekdays in the city with George. We'd pig out at Red Lobster, the two of us, no doubt looking like an odd pair: George, a short, distinguished man in his golden years, with thinning hair and slight moustache; and me, a young, very pregnant woman wearing a wedding ring. He often pretended to be my sugar daddy, getting laughs from our good-humored waiters. I loved his sense of humor and wisdom. Despite the fact that he'd lived a long and wonderful life, losing him was another blow in a crappy string of sad stories.

I could see and feel two clichés vying for time within me: "Bad things happen in threes" was taking center stage, but, "Live every day like it's your last," gained momentum as well. In other words, I was tired of feeling like a victim, so I thought I could flip the script and do something different. How about a vacation from all these worried thoughts?

After rapid research, I booked a trip to the Dominican Republic. With what seemed like light speed, I found myself packing. We had never traveled anywhere with our children, so I was careful to get advice from our doctor on international travel, which included multiple vaccinations, mostly for Emma – injections she despised. She was due for her second MMR (measles, mumps and rubella) at this time, plus a second shot for her first year of flu vaccine. She qualified for the chicken pox vaccine, hepatitis A, oh – and malaria pills, so I went along with doctor's orders.

God, it all seems so obvious now, but being a trusting medical technologist, I followed the advice I was given to a tee – crossing each shot off my list, all within the same week. I ignored the little voice inside my head asking how it could possibly be okay to bombard my daughter's body with so much immune-manipulating mayhem. Our son got off easier with just the hepatitis A shot and flu booster.

Medically topped up, we prepared our luggage to leave the country. As we loaded the car for our six-hour trip to the airport hotel, Will, who had attended his buddy Jake's birthday party the night before, felt sick to his stomach and began vomiting. Just like that. One minute he was gathering toys for the car and the next minute he was puking all over the kitchen floor.

"Cancel the trip, Jules," warned the little voice in my head. The words came through loud and clear, just as they did when Emma grimaced through her immunizations. But the car was packed, the trip already paid for. *Perhaps it's just some fluke of nerves or excited vomit, if there is such a thing.*

Anxious, we phoned friends and family for advice, mostly looking for support to find a way to *go* on our exotic foreign escapade. Successfully convinced that kids frequently get stomach upsets (although ours never had), we soldiered on.

If only I'd been open to something radical, like changing my plans. If only I'd been more observant to the message my wonderfully intuitive son was sending us, a message that screamed: *Hey, I'm young and sick and can dehydrate easily. How about we use our insurance coverage to cancel this trip for another time, because ... by the way ... something BAD is going to happen on OUR FLIGHT!*

Did I heed this generous signal from the universe to stay home and postpone flying halfway around the world for another time? Nope. Did I listen to my internal guidance system? I wish. Sadly, once again, I ignored my gut instincts and obvious cues because it would be highly inconvenient to do otherwise. I may as well have been unconscious, focusing solely on the future we *should* have instead of accepting the events of the moment.

Onward we went with our barfing three-year-old, stopping several times along the way to empty his sick bucket and comfort him back into his medicated sleep.

By the next morning Will's barfing had passed, just as our friends said it would.

Perhaps I'd overreacted. I really should loosen up.

With a deep breath of relief, Marc and I boarded the plane with our children.

The flight itself was uneventful. We played games with Emma, and Will slept. When we began our descent, Emma wanted to know the logistics of landing a plane, which Marc explained.

"It's so much safer than traveling in a car. Landing is a piece of cake. Just remember to keep swallowing like on the way up to keep your ears from feeling funny."

I smiled, looking over at my beautiful family. How lucky I was to be blessed with my husband, a fantastic father, and my adorable, delightful brood. I was excited at the prospect of playing in the ocean with them – uninterrupted quality time together ... *finally*.

The plane approached the ground quickly. Marc looked at me with a strange expression, which worried me because he's a frequent flyer. Then came a moment no one can prepare for. Time literally slowed to a snail's pace when the plane *smashed* onto the runway. We rebounded back into the air with a horrifying jolt of force, our heads whipping forward. The plane seemed to tilt slightly to one side and plunged back to the ground, smashing us onto the runway again. Overhead compartments broke open, their contents flying throughout the cabin. We were out of control and still traveling at an incredible rate of speed. To my right, a TV screen came loose from the ceiling, I instinctively reached around to my left to protect Emma. The plane smashed down a third time with a force so strong it jarred my twisted back the wrong way, causing me to lose my breath. *Is this really happening?*

I wish I could tell you I embraced this moment with the intent of meeting my maker with a peaceful heart. Hell no, I'm no yogi. Rather than being ready to surrender to the will of God, I was a mother lion protecting her cubs and clinging to SURVIVAL. As Marc and I grabbed onto our precious children I was suddenly flooded with remorse. *Oh, my god ... I've just killed my family!*

I believed this totally. Like a snapshot of my entire life, I saw how I'd ruined everything. The trip was *all* my idea. I'd pushed ahead, despite my son's imperative message to delay our travels. And here we were. What had I been thinking? Where was my brain?

I looked up from my seat to see everyone around me clutching whatever or whomever they could, and wondered how this would unfold.

Would a fireball come careening toward us after the plane ran off the runway and crashed into something? Would the final impact crush us? Would my children suffer, or would this be quick? Where were the exits? Did we all have our shoes on? Would they even stay on?

These thoughts flew through my neurons faster than the speed of light, adrenal glands on maximum thrust. The fight-or-flight response made me ready to do whatever was necessary to live – the almighty, genetically built-in, primal desire to stay alive.

Then, just as quickly as the episode began, our plane managed to stop. Dazed, we all looked around in disbelief. The smell of jet fuel hung in the air, alerting us to the urgency of getting off the plane NOW! The attendants scrambled to open crumpled doors that wouldn't budge. TV screens still dangled from walls and oxygen masks hung like marionettes.

Will and Emma were unusually quiet and compliant as I comforted them. Ignoring the pain in my back, I focused solely on protecting my children and getting them off that plane.

Marc grabbed our bags and cleared the way for us into the aisle. Finally, the front door of the plane opened and we eagerly filed into the humid Caribbean night.

Darkness oozed toward us from the tropical atmosphere, the thick, salty, warm air rushing into our lungs. Palm trees and exotic critters moved in the shadows. Although we couldn't see the landscape, there was an instant feeling of being in another country.

The airport staff and emergency crew surrounded our plane with wide-eyed awe on their faces as they surveyed the damage and whispered to one another in Spanish. The plane was literally creased through the middle, bent like a toy just in front of where we had been sitting. Yet, somehow, we were all walking off. How does something like this happen?

The crew, realizing the damaged engines still posed a fire threat, directed us toward the terminal like dazed cattle and then herded us off to our respective hotels on tourist buses.

I cringed with back pain as we bumped over the primitive roads and was relieved to reach our hotel; however, my relief was short lived, because Will started vomiting again. This time, between the heat and his already dehydrated state, he deteriorated quickly. The next morning we saw the hotel doctor, who sent us to the tourist hospital by ambulance, where Will spent two days on intravenous fluids. I stayed with him while Marc and Emma tried to enjoy the beach at our hotel. At least the hospital was nice, done up exclusively for unfortunate tourists like us. I was grateful to have a bed in the hospital next to Will so I could rest my back.

On day three we returned to the hotel to join Marc and Emma, only to face dire complications. Will now had severe diarrhea. Back to the hospital we went, over the tortuous, pothole-ridden Dominican roads.

On day six of our seven-day trip, we managed to get back to our hotel, but it was now Emma's turn to get sick to *her* stomach. Fearing dehydration during our long journey home, Emma and I checked back into the hospital where she was hooked up to an I.V. for twenty-four hours until it was time to board a plane to fly home (the thought of which, by the way, left me petrified).

I had spent an entire week in a hospital tending my children and my back, and then I had to face the prospect of getting on a plane to go home. Oh, and shall I mention the complete anxiety attack (a real one) during the flight; my flare-up of inflammatory bowel issues that hung on for months afterwards; and my accompanying back pain and sleeping troubles? And I certainly can't leave out Will's newly acquired eczema. The poor little guy was covered by a rash. Need I go on ... blah-blah-blah...

It was official: I was now a *crap magnet*! I was completely caught up in helplessness and fear. I was stuck on my trauma train with no clue how to get off. If only I could have focused on the things that really mattered in life, all the good that still surrounded me, even amid the chaos. My negative vibration kept me blinded, like straining to see through mud. I couldn't appreciate the joyful facts of my brother-in-law's safe return from Bangkok, the treasured opportunity to be with my best friend before she left this world, or the fact that we miraculously survived a potentially deadly plane crash.

Something about an ever-present, seemingly invisible disease can remind one of the preciousness of every moment, the glory of being here every day, every minute. This lesson was ultimately provided by my beautiful, brave daughter. Emma was about to become sick, and our lives would never be the same.

Chapter 8

The Yellow Brick Road

Back to 2007 ~ August

CAW, CAW, RINGS THROUGH THE AIR like a scene from a scary movie. Menacing black crows flap their wings at the fluffy intruder approaching their prized nest. With towels wrapped around our dripping swimsuits, we scramble to the cool shade of the tallest tree in our yard. "Please come down!" we plead.

This is the third tree Mojo has climbed in as many weeks. She's still young and the thrill of reaching the top of a tall, bramble-ridden conifer hasn't worn off. Intent on reaching the bird nest, she flattens out as much as she can, trying to make herself undetectable, unfazed by the angry crows circling above.

Mojo squeaks out that hunter meow – the kind felines produce when they've trapped a fly on the window ledge. With the primal instincts of a panther raging through her, she dares the birds to come closer. *Oh, to have a mouth full of those black feathers!*

Emma and Will do not share her excitement. They're crying. "Mommy, Mommy, they're going to eat her. We have to get her down!"

I sigh and head for the garage to get the ladder. This time Mojo has climbed an old, prickly, blue spruce tree, and I can only work the ladder into the first row of dense branches. She's far out of reach. Even if I were brave enough to go that high, I couldn't.

"That's it, I've had it," I declare. "I can't keep risking my neck to get that ridiculous cat out of trees. We'll just have to leave her there. Maybe she'll finally learn her lesson."

"No, no, no! You can't! No, Mommy, no!"

I slump to the ground and bury my head in my hands. "Even if Daddy *were* home, he wouldn't be able to reach her like he did before. She'll eventually come down on her own. There's nothing I can do this time."

The crows grow increasingly agitated, jumping onto different branches, moving closer to our beloved Mojo. Perhaps they're starting to realize the odds are in their favor.

"What about a fireman, Mommy?" Emma asks. "They always save kitties in trees, don't they?"

I take in several more breaths to calm my anxiety. I can no more leave Mojo in that tree than they can. I don't know why I would say otherwise.

What could it hurt, other than my pride, to call a fireman? We see this all the time in cartoons, so there must be some sort of truth in it – I hope. With my cell phone I dial 911. This is *so* ridiculous; they'll laugh at me for sure. Or worse, I'll get a fine for being a prank caller. Maybe I should hang up. *Crap,* they have call display, they'll just track me down anyway. It's too late...

"What is the nature of your emergency, please?" the operator asks.

"Uh, well..." I stall, as I begin to consider my apology for pushing the wrong button.

"Ma'am?"

"I'm very sorry," I start. I've never been a good fabricator of untruths ... here goes nothing. "I'm very sorry if I'm wasting your time, but I ... ahh ... well ... my kitten is stuck at the top of a very tall tree, and she can't come down. A couple of angry crows are looking to make lunch out of her, and I fear my children are going need years of expensive therapy if I don't figure out how to get her down fairly soon."

"You have a cat stuck in a tree?" the operator coldly confirms.

Completely embarrassed to waste the time of emergency services on a ***non-human*** emergency, I respond, "Yes."

"Sounds like you need the fire department, Ma'am. I'll put you through."

Surprised and hoping I might not be entirely crazy, I wait for the voice of our volunteer fire chief to come on the line. I repeat my dilemma, this time with a little more confidence. I finish with a nervous laugh as visions of a shiny red fire engine pulling up to our yard form in my mind, complete with our neighbors circled around, and Will's eyes as large as basketballs.

The fire chief pulls up to our house, cell phone still to his ear. No shiny red truck, but there he is, just like that. He gets out and stands at the bottom of the tree, contemplating his options. Before I can contribute to the rescue plan, he has his jacket off and is at the top of my ladder calling to Mojo. Emma and Will jump up and down, trying to convince her to go to the nice fireman. But she can't; she's pretty much stuck about ten feet beyond the reach of the ladder.

"Would one of your truck ladders be able to get up there?" I ask, pushing the limits of my bold request for help.

"No, this tree is too thick," he says. Then, with a decisive look on his face, he begins to climb the tree, free hand: no ladder, no ropes, no safety net. He climbs higher and higher, scraping himself on the rough, jagged spears filling out the tree's interior. I can't look. I'm terrified he'll fall, all because of my numbskull cat. Emma and Will squeal with joy and apprehension as this courageous man risks his neck for our precious baby.

Mojo sizes up her rescuer and projects a casual meow at him as he reaches up with one hand and grabs her. She's not afraid of him; she becomes limp and relaxed, resistance free, making it easier for this heroic man to navigate back down. I reach for her and pull her in tight, like the first day I found her at the shelter. She looks up at me with those talking eyes.

"See, no big deal. All you had to do was ask for help, silly. What was so hard about that?"

Our Most Difficult First Year with Diabetes ~ 2006

If only I had Mojo's wisdom during our first year with diabetes, a time when I felt so alone and needed to ask for help most of all. Even Dorothy had enough brains to do this when she started on her journey down the yellow brick road. I wish I'd been one of those people you hear about who wakes up one day with a completely enlightened perspective after a life-altering experience – calm, serene, all knowing. Yeah. Hardly.

2005 was a year filled with life-altering whammies: the tsunami, Karen's death, our crash landing. Then, six months later we ended the year with Emma's diagnosis only two weeks before Christmas. You'd think I'd start 2006 with a new clarity on life, but instead I had to focus on my new job as a pancreas. Since Astrid found other employment quickly, I was back to my usual line up of helpers: *No one.*

This meant adjustments within our lives fell predominately upon me, as Marc was away eighty-five percent of the time. I had no option but to tough it out, which made our survival all consuming.

Struggle number one was to figure out why Emma's blood sugars would never behave the same way more than twice. In an effort to understand her body, I created color-coded excel spreadsheets and sliding-scale carb and insulin grids. I read every book I could get my hands on, and Googled daily to find some shred of evidence that this disease would be cured somehow, and soon. I seriously considered applying for a job at Emma's school. I spent so much time there anyway – educating the other teachers, being available for extracurricular activities, arranging conference call meetings with my pediatrician, the principal, secretaries, educational assistants. It took a Herculean effort to set up new policies and protocols on handling a newly diagnosed, unstable, seven-year-old, type 1 diabetic.

The harsh reality of Emma's condition was that she required my constant, undivided attention nearly all the time. My sweet, deeply concerned son had to take a back seat far too often during my dramatic battles with Emma, as she would constantly resist her needles or refuse to finish meals for which she had already taken insulin. I often saw Will anxiously pace the floors, concerned for Emma's ordeal, wondering if she would survive her next injection.

Besides that, mood changes accompanied Emma's blood sugar swings. I swear, the first time she had a low blood sugar I felt like I was watching Linda Blair in *The Exorcist*. Emma's voice deepened, and she became completely enraged, almost growling at us. We were so distraught by her radical character transformation and refusal to drink a juice to bring her blood sugar back up, that we rushed her to the ER, trying to coax a straight shooter of sugar into her mouth the whole way. She just looked at me through her eyebrows mumbling lines from *The Shining* and *Dirty Harry*:

"Redrum ... Redrum. Do you feel lucky punk?" Or something equally crazy. Luckily for us, the nurse on duty had a son with type 1 diabetes, and she gently guided us through our first rookie panic attack.

We were supposed to be in what they call the honeymoon phase, where there's still some function of insulin producing cells, thus making blood sugars more stable. If this was a honeymoon, I wanted our money back. The slightest change of food or insulin created dramatic swings in her blood sugar levels. When she was happy and having fun, her blood sugars were at their best. If she felt angry, stressed, or bored, her blood sugars were at their worst. Cold days – blood sugars go up. Hot days – blood sugars go down. Illness or growth spurts – they go up. Exercise, nervousness, or excitement – they go down. Even a hot bath could bring them dangerously low. I worked endlessly to try and find some sort of balance, but there *was* no balance, only intense effort and dedication to keep up.

Six months post-diagnosis, we graduated from injections to an insulin pump, an incredible device that allows a person to control insulin, similar to an actual pancreas. This proved more effective than injections, as it allowed for much smaller doses of insulin. A pump is attached by a narrow plastic tube called a cannula, which is inserted with the help of a needle, into the abdomen, bum or thigh regions. The needle is then removed leaving the narrow cannula under the skin. The pump itself looks a lot like a waist belt pager, attached at all times to the body at the infusion site, with a new site required approximately every three days.

The best part of the pump is the ability to inject insulin on the spot or "bolus" when eating a carbohydrate meal. This allowed Emma to have more freedom over what she wanted to eat and when. If her classmates at school were having a treat outside the scheduled lunch break, we could handle that. Our life of rigid meal times and schedules improved dramatically, as we could now make small, subtle changes with her insulin as often as needed.

But we had much more reason to be vigilant now, with more potential complications, the need to stay one-step ahead of the mechanics of the pump itself, and monitoring reliability of the infusion sites. My night shifts were always the favorite time for an infusion site to stop infusing properly, air to enter the tubing line, or mysterious high blood sugars to sleuth out. I had to act quickly. For diabetics on a pump, a blood sugar level should not remain high for more than four hours, as DKA can occur quickly, which again, is life threatening.

Technical jargon became a new reality of our life. This reality would have me up four or five times a night, providing many opportunities to phone our on-call endocrinologist at 3:00 a.m., asking what to do next. This reality would bring an ambulance to our house at 6:00 a.m. after a night of trying to stabilize Emma's blood sugar, which could be thrown into turmoil by a simple stomach flu. My constant goal was to keep her from falling into a coma.

In an amplified way, this was similar to bringing Emma home after she was born. All of a sudden, someone's life depended on *me* knowing what to do. All of a sudden, I no longer slept through the night, and my needs were not a priority. Everything was about this incredible, beautiful child who had miraculously formed within my own body – a child I would do *anything* for, take on a thousand sleepless nights if I had to, just from the enormity of my love for her.

But Emma would not be outgrowing the cause of my concern anytime soon. There was no cure for what ailed her. *Yet.*

~ ~ ~ ~

During that difficult first year I increasingly learned to trust my instincts on what to do, rather than rely on my charts and grids (which is a difficult thing to teach others). I became acutely aware of how Emma's body worked. I could often tell she was getting sick before she knew it herself, simply by what her blood sugars were doing. I could detect a subtle odor on her breath when she had high blood sugars – a sort of sweet sore-throat smell. Now I can pick up that scent from several feet away, like a well-trained bloodhound. Then there's a look she gets when her blood sugar is low – like a grey fog surrounding her eyes.

My learning seemed endless, the lack of sleep, *excruciating*. All I wanted for Emma was a normal childhood. I did everything I could to achieve this. The result was my complete and utter exhaustion: physical, mental, and financial.

~ ~ ~ ~

On a cool, rainy, October evening ten months into our diabetic life, Marc was cleaning up the last of the dishes from dinner as I began gathering the supplies needed for Emma's site change. As Marc placed the final dish into the drying rack, he casually glanced at me from the kitchen sink.

"We need to face reality, Julie. Bad things happen; that's just the way life is. We can't keep dreaming everything will work out. We need to put the house up for sale." He paused for a moment and then made a move toward the door. "Can you start making a list of what we need to do while I'm away this week? We'll deal with this when I get back."

Thankfully, Emma and Will were in another room. The look on my face might have brought them to tears. Yes, I knew this moment would come, but I'd been successful at hiding from it during the past ten months, like an ostrich plunging its head into soft sand. Marc's words caught me completely off guard.

I sat there in disbelief, my mouth open, grasping for something clever to say as visions of us struggling to make ends meet flooded my mind. Surely we could find a way to avoid this calamity. Good always wins in the end, doesn't it?

Perhaps I was delusional to think I could achieve a better existence for myself when I'd stared hopefully at the TV screen from beneath Chicken Grammy's arm. After everything that happened since the tsunami, perhaps Marc was actually right. Maybe life *was* meant to be hard. Maybe my future would be nothing more than learning to survive as a dead-tired walking zombie.

Numb and defeated, I couldn't think of a single reason to *not* sell. Our house had required loads of sweat equity over the past five years. Maybe it *was* too big for me to handle, especially with Marc gone so much: the in-ground concrete pool, the elaborate gardens surrounding our interlocking brick deck, the inevitable repairs required every spring after the ravages of long, cold, snowy winters.

But hold on ... I love it here. I love being within a five-minute walk to school, to the stores, to the beach. I don't want to go back to a small house like our first home – a home so tiny you needed to go outside just to change your mind.

I truly wasn't ready to give up more than we already had.

Realistically, I knew we had to make plans to sell, yet the reality of it crushed me more than I could have expected. This was only a house, right? But because I was so bloody tired, it felt like the end of the rest of my world.

That night Marc and I barely spoke. Tension followed us like a cloud of dense fog. Since diabetes penetrated our family, neither of us had been able to discuss our true feelings – the disappointments and the fear. For Marc, I suspect he was uncomfortable with what seemed like my abandonment as a financial contributor. But being a pancreas was a 24/7 job; I had nothing left to offer toward my hard-earned career in ultrasound. And because he was away so much, he couldn't keep up with Emma's changing needs, including the refusal on her part to have anyone but me do her needles (not at all a wise trend).

Being on my own so much, I developed an independence and self-sufficiency to survive. Regrettably, every time Marc returned home it became more difficult to incorporate him back into our routines. He seemed to only notice the things I didn't get done while he was away.

"You missed garbage day," or, "There's an inch of dust on this window ledge."

But what about all the things I did do, like keeping Emma and Will alive this week on almost no sleep? And so enters the proverbial elephant, sitting in the middle of our living room.

Communication between Marc and I began feeling like fingernails on a chalkboard. Marc's all-consuming job and a child with all-consuming needs pushed us beyond our already inadequate coping skills.

When the sun rose the following morning I began making notes on what we needed to do before listing our house. I wanted so much to believe we could make adjustments somewhere else, but with my vitality and energy a distant memory, I couldn't see how. I knew life could be so much more difficult than this. There are far worse conditions for children to suffer. What nerve did I have to feel so defeated, so broken down? My only answer to this now is ... sleep deprivation, a most effective form of torture.

Marc headed off to the airport while I got Emma and Will to school. I returned home to a quiet house and opened my notebook, staring blankly at the letters scratched onto the page. Maybe I should start with something easier, I thought, as I dragged myself to the basement in search of a friendly pile of laundry.

I scanned our large family room: toys not put away, clothes that needed folding, the tumbling sounds of wet towels in the dryer. I flopped down on Uncle George's favorite floral sofa – the one he bequeathed to me before he passed away – my mind a complete void. I gazed blankly at the ceiling. Was this it? Was this what life would turn out to be, just a crazy test of endurance?

I was surrounded by emptiness, with no visible way out. No family around to give me a break and no money to pay someone to help. No one seemed to understand what it was like: the day-in and day-out impossibility of being the one in control of a little girl's blood sugar every second of her existence. This situation held no room for slacking; Emma's very life depended on *me*.

I'd been told that in time we would adjust to our new lifestyle and it would feel normal, as long as I made sure I wasn't the sole person to tend to Emma's needs. But despite the doctors' warnings to avoid this onerous task alone, I was the only one available to do it.

I lay there in the silence, overcome by an intense aching in my heart. The feeling worked its way up into my throat, as often happened in the past. But this time, instead of holding back, I let the feelings escape. Like a waterfall of pent up sorrow, my tears began flowing, soft at first, weak and weary. Then deeper, lower, until the sobs vibrated within my chest. These were tears that seemed to have no end, tears I should have shed long ago but suppressed for the sake of my family. I had tried to stay strong, but it was official – I was anything but. I needed to find a way out of the dark hole I had fallen into, but I also needed a sign, a rope, a neon light pointing the way out. I finally cried for help to whoever could hear me. God ... Karen ... Uncle George. I begged out loud to that outer zone, the concealed mystical world beyond my shielded vision.

I blubbered, "Show me how to turn things around, please, *I NEED HELP!*"

I felt for the first time how a person could become so lost that nothing made sense anymore. I knew how it felt to be desperately tired and ready to pack it in – call it quits and try again in another lifetime perhaps, because I had definitely screwed this one up, big time.

I lay in the silence until I fell asleep – exhausted and completely drained. Then the timer on the dryer buzzed.

Who would do the laundry if I wasn't here? I thought as I awoke from my groggy state, the warm fluffy towels pulling me from my gloom and back to the reality of life – a life I would soon learn was only hours away from radically transforming – a life I knew needed to change. But I didn't know how to make that first step (or rather, that first flat-out stumble and fall).

Until now.

Complex equations, medical texts, and spreadsheets weren't going to help me. The very act of asking the unseen world for guidance – the act of trusting in a place no one can prove exists – was the beginning of my yellow brick road. I needed to abandon my limited belief systems, lower my resistance, and *ask for help*. Help, I have since learned, WILL come every time, with no exceptions. I just need to stay open to it.

"No big deal silly. What was so hard about that?"

Part 2

When you change the way you look at things...
the things you look at change.

~ Dr. Wayne Dyer

Chapter 9

Over the Rainbow

A FRAGRANT BREEZE SATURATES the air, filling my senses with lavender, rosehip, and tea tree. The effect is immediate – calm and comforting, like snuggling in a soft, warm blanket wrapped in the arms of someone I love.

I feel no more fear of the unknown, only excitement. No more striving to fit in, only acceptance. No more facades to put on, only humility and honesty. This place can be anywhere and still feel like home. Welcome to the magical, alluring land of spirituality, just Over the Rainbow – a place that can appear when storm clouds part and life-sustaining rays of the sun illuminate the crisp, clean atmosphere. All the colors separate for a brief moment to reveal their secrets, then come together to create pure, white light.

This is what humans seek, what we can achieve when we realize we are not separate. When we join in unity, purpose, and love, we reclaim our true radiance. We are spiritually connected beings. We're all the different colors of the rainbow, and together *we are* pure, white light.

This is how spirituality feels to me: a glimpse of forest through the trees. For a few blissful moments I know life contains more than strife. I recognize, at last, how many joyous things await me, the divine grace of every action I take, the purpose of my existence. Then the veil moves in again, and centuries of genetic programming pull me back to my primitive nature.

Embracing a spiritual life has been challenging for me, with a taste here, a kick in the pants there. The inherent peace isn't something that stayed with me once I sampled it. What would be the fun in that? My quest for the spiritual has been an adventure, a journey, sometimes a game of cat and mouse. Just when I begin to feel more enlightened a new challenge flies into my life, bringing opportunities for more growth and deeper awareness.

Some see a spiritual life as cult-like, addictive, even woo-woo. And let's face it; some of it does walk that line. To discern between cult and spirituality, let's look at the meaning of these words:

Cult: *Followers of an exclusive system of beliefs and practices. An interest followed with exaggerated zeal; followers of an unorthodox, extremist, or organized false-religion or sect who often live outside of conventional society under the direction of a charismatic leader, causing harm.*

Does spirituality follow this definition?

Spirituality: *Can refer to an ultimate or immaterial reality – an inner path enabling a person to discover the essence of being, or the deepest values and meanings by which people live. Spiritual practices, including meditation, prayer, and contemplation, are intended to develop an individual's inner life. Such practices often lead to an experience of connectedness with a larger reality, yielding a more comprehensive self – with other individuals or the human community, with nature or the cosmos, or with the devine realm. Spirituality is often experienced as a source of inspiration or orientation in life. It can encompass belief in immaterial realities or experiences of the immanent or transcendent nature of the world.*

To me, the critical words isolating the term cult are "causing harm," whereas spirituality is about "source inspiration and connectedness to all life."

I have no doubt the spiritual realm is different and mystical. In a spiritual world anything seems possible: fairies, angels, multidimensional enlightened teachers from the Great Beyond, extraterrestrials, crystals that vibrate healing energy, vortexes, and levitation. Here we find a kingdom filled with unexplained beauty, history, and ritual: the pyramids, the lost cities of Atlantis and Lemuria, Machu Picchu, sweat lodges, sacred ceremonies, geometric shapes, crystal bowls, and gongs. Of course we can't leave out the allure of incense, candles, meditation, prayers, Tai Chi, Chi Gong, yoga, chakras, empathetics, psychics, clairsentients, clairvoyants, healers, mystics, raw foodists, vegetarians and astrologers. On and on I can go, with no end to the variations. All these different names, rules, and teachers are striving for the same outcome – to achieve balance within the body and mind while connected to spirit and our source energy. This good juju, if you will, is meant to help us fulfill our goals and our destiny.

If the goal is to help, provide love and guidance, and cause *no* harm, then I feel safe on my non-cult side of the line.

Extreme interpretations and charlatans can give spirituality a bad rap. And surely, some of it *is* a freak show, or at least bizarre. Nevertheless, how can I deny the experiences of others and only accept my own as real? Just because something doesn't seem true to me doesn't mean it's not true for someone else.

Belief is the result of personal experience, and every person on this planet has different experiences. Therein lies the confusion.

While on an Alaskan cruise I saw an exceptionally funny comedian who hilariously described our boat as being filled with magical spiritual folk (or wizards, like in *Harry Potter*). The boat trailing us was, in her words, filled with "regular, everyday, non-magical folks – aka, *Muggles*." My kids and I are big *Harry Potter* fans, so this description felt accurate in an amusing way.

Since I jumped into the more esoteric spiritual practices, I've often felt like a timid Muggle in a magical world. I still get caught up in my left-brained rational mind while trying to open my spirit to the limitless possibilities of the universe. If only I could pull a

Liz Gilbert and take a year off in my seeking. Maybe then I'd have the time and presence of mind to make more sense of it.

But wait a minute. I'm a mom living in the mainstream world. If I truly believe in this sort of thing, then I must admit I chose my path for this lifetime. I need to skip the ashrams for now and try the truest test of awakening – a test that keeps me firmly entrenched in the "real" world, with my children as my greatest teachers.

What I will now attempt to describe is *my* experience, one that feels real to me because I am the person living it – an experience I put through my own filters of belief, allowing my inner guidance to lead the way.

October 2006

The day after my basement plea for help, things began happening. With my resistance down and my heart finally cracked open from the release of suffocating sadness, I began to notice occurrences and coincidences. I felt as though I'd finally closed my umbrella and let the rain reach me. At last, the cascading, limitless, purifying water of help that had always been around me was now becoming visible.

Since the plane incident, my back required regular care to keep it from going out. I went to visit my friend and massage therapist (I'll call her Lisa) for my weekly appointment. We discussed the usual topics – the kids, my pain, and fatigue – before our conversation turned to a movie she'd just received from one of her clients.

"It's an interesting movie," she said. "I watched it last night. I can't describe what it's about, except to say I'm almost sure you'll like it. Would you like to borrow it?"

Watching movies is something I've always enjoyed and the one thing I could manage with my low energy, so I took it home.

Once I cleaned up dinner and got homework and baths out of the way, I asked the kids if they wanted to watch with me. Lisa had given it the "suitable-for-children" green light. This wasn't the kind of movie they would normally see, but it contained no harmful violence, sex, or swearing. With no clue to its content and Marc away for the better part of two weeks, the kids and I settled in front of the big screen and pushed play.

The show drew us in right from the beginning. Even Emma and Will were getting into it, which surprised me because this was a group of grownups talking about a universal force called *the Law of Attraction*. They discussed being magnificent creators of their own lives, in a "magical genie" sort of way – able to cure diseases and be one with the universe.

I was glued to the TV by this perfectly timed movie called *The Secret* – a fusion of science, like a *Quantum Physics for Dummies* tutorial. The common sense was so profound, yet simple. Somewhere deep down I felt a stirring of awareness, an intense knowing, like when I met Marc or saw Mojo for the first time.

When the movie ended Emma and Will went into high gear, as if they'd eaten too much candy. Skipping and jumping around, giggling and playing – in no state for going to bed any time soon. I, on the other hand, sat there in complete silence, stunned. Just yesterday I had broken down and asked the unknown for help. Now, here I was in my own living room watching a movie that discussed the laws of the universe and how to use them to improve my life; a movie that explained how the very thoughts and feelings I choose today will attract the experiences I have in my future.

Just when I was ready to give up on my grand notions of living a magnificent life, here was a neon sign in my greatest moment of need. My plea for help *must* have been heard. Chills ran up and down my spine as I felt the presence of something bigger than myself gently grab my hand and help me off the couch.

In a light-bulb moment of simplicity, I felt euphoric and relieved to see how I'd been swept so far off track. All I needed to do was reprogram my thoughts and my vibrations, my signals to the universe.

For the past two years I'd been locked into the devastation or "vibration" that began with the tsunami and images of that frightened, traumatized boy. If quantum physics *was* valid, then I was unknowingly responsible, or at least a serious co-creator, for how I experienced the events that came into my life. My thoughts had matched and amplified the original signals I sent out the day of the tsunami.

Quantum physics says we can live many possible realities at any given moment, that the observer influences the actual outcome of an experience. I don't believe we can actually change a particular event, but we can affect the way we perceive it.

This made so much sense. All the drama of the past two years carried identical feelings: helplessness, fear of death, and forces beyond my control. These feelings became larger and more extreme with each event. I was a textbook case. I was responsible for becoming a crap magnet and the good news was – according to the theme of this movie – "whatever we do can be undone." I could turn things around!

This message was like a life-vest thrown into the hands of my overboard, sinking self. I finally had tools! I watched the film several more times and shared it with my friends and family. Two days later I received an invitation from three different people to attend a Law of Attraction workshop.

Then, Amazon.com sent me a routine advertisement about a book for balancing the body's internal ecosystem, *The Body Ecology Diet* by Donna Gates. I bought it, just like that. The information I needed began to follow me around, whispering in my ear and tapping me on the shoulder. I believe it had always been there, but I was too closed off to notice.

My eyes were wide open for the first time, like moving from a black and white world into a Technicolor life filled with strange-looking new people, beautiful fresh fragrances, scenery, and friends – great new quirky, spiritual friends. *Non-Muggles* to be exact, who seemed to love me, flaws and all, and accept me without judgment.

They didn't call me crazy for hoping Emma could be cured. In fact, they didn't see any good reason why not. I felt as if the doors had opened to allow angels into my life. I suspect these angels follow some kind of rule, like *they can only come in when invited.* So I invited them in. Tardy but enthusiastic, I began my journey down the yellow brick road, located in a new and colorful world on the other side of the rainbow. I would believe in this Oz place again, the one that captured my imagination so many years ago as I snuggled beneath Chicken Grammy's arm. In this place, miracles *can* and *do* happen.

And maybe, just maybe, they could happen for us.

Chapter 10

A New Brain

November 2006

USING SUGGESTIONS FROM *The Secret*, I started to work immediately. Like a hungry miner searching for the last vestiges of gold, I left no stone unturned. I began studying Feng Shui, the ancient Chinese system of aesthetics. I learned ways to harness the laws of both Heaven (through astronomy) and Earth (through geography) to radically improve life by tapping into positive "qi" or energy.

Needless to say, I rearranged everything – the entire house. I drew a map of our home, searching for the most auspicious alignment of energy based on each family member's birth date. I then got out the compass and spun beds around, hung chimes in the right places, and softened sharp corners with plants and furniture. I was prepared to learn Chinese if it would help; I was that determined.

Belief is an important component of Feng Shui – belief in good luck versus bad luck. I loved the idea of thinking thoughts of fostering GOOD luck for a change, thoughts that weren't related to blood sugars, natural disasters, or plane crashes. My mind enjoyed having something new to play with. As I no longer desired to dwell on anything "bad," I concerned myself mostly with the good-luck aspects of Feng Shui. I trusted the validity of these respected and ancient Chinese traditions, and handed myself over completely to the process.

I realized belief is the key for *any* form of ritualistic behavior. From black cats, four leaf clovers, broken mirrors, shooting stars, Friday the 13th, lucky rabbit's feet, to walking under ladders. If you believe something brings good luck or bad luck, it will.

Our post office box number at this time was 1313 – a number often associated with rotten luck. At the time we received the number I made a conscious decision I didn't believe in bad luck omens. However, after the year we'd just endured I was willing to entertain any idea that could change our fortune, just in case. Imagine my delight when I enquired about changing our P.O. Box and was offered box number 77. Seven is my favorite number.

"I'll take it," I sang.

I continued posting images throughout the house to reflect excellent health, adventure, financial security, and joy. Our entire home became my vision board, each wall my canvas. I'd stick reminders on the bathroom mirror and on the fridge, with art on our walls that made me feel good. Every room demonstrated something I hoped to attract into our lives. Mostly I managed to keep my efforts unobtrusive, blending into the décor.

Marc noticed the changes I made, and while he wasn't necessarily on board, he didn't object either. Deep down, I think he was much more accepting of my efforts than I gave him credit for, despite his less than enthusiastic input.

One night over dinner I probed each family member to give specific details toward creating the perfect family holiday. Marc's contribution to the conversation was a glorious, glaring, stink eye that screamed, *Why are you entertaining such ridiculous ideas? We have no money for stupid pipe dreams!* However, what he actually said was, "When the money starts pouring in and we no longer have financial worries, I'll be on board with you." This left me with a large rabbit to pull from my new faith fedora.

Next, I needed to get rid of clutter. With this I was ruthless. Clutter had to go, whether in the closets, corners, our files, or in storage. Our living space needed to be reamed out and cleaned out. I became obsessed with creating space and energy flow for new and better things to come into our lives. It felt wonderful to give bags of old toys and clothes to the Diabetes Clothesline. Not only were we improving the look and energy of our home, we also were able to contribute toward the Canadian Diabetes Association, another step in the right direction.

The Rewind Game was my next creation, a game my children were keen to play, *at first.* Anytime someone verbalized what he or she did *not* want, we would shout, "Push the rewind button!" and then say the opposite. I was amazed how often we said what we didn't want, such as, "If you don't hurry up, we'll be late." I said this all the time, and guess what? We were always late for *everything*! When we pushed the rewind button, we would follow up with, "We have lots of time."

Emma and Will were quick learners and kept me on my toes anytime I said something negative, which was often. This game brought an acute awareness of how frequently we focused on what we didn't want. But it was only fun for the kids when they could catch and torture someone else for "being negative." No one liked being the one actually caught.

"Will, you're so annoying," was Emma's most popular phrase.

"Will, you're such a *great* brother," Will would sing back with a smirk, knowing I would back him up on that rewind.

"No way. Not happening!" Emma would say as she crossed her arms in stubborn defiance.

...Well, it was mostly a good game, for a little while. At least my heart was in the right place.

I then put my focus on a particular quote from *The Secret*, which stated, "The way you feel is everything." I began searching my mental archives for the times in my life when I felt invincible. It seemed obvious to me that generating feelings of joy and happiness would be instrumental in changing the frequency I had been emitting since becoming obsessed with all-things tragic.

On a hunch during a night when Emma's blood sugars were not cooperating, I thought to search through my old photo albums and keepsake boxes. Choosing to stay up rather than force myself to wake up again in an hour's time seemed like a smart thing to do. As I was feeling a tad sorry for myself as well, this felt like a perfect opportunity to shift my thoughts to more pleasant times.

Curled up with my favorite blanket and a warm cup of Sleepy Time tea in front of a fire still glowing within the woodstove, I began searching through our collection of baby albums and wedding photos. Within a few minutes I reached for the New Zealand album, a book documenting the seven-month adventure I'd taken nearly ten years earlier. What better place to start my quest than a land filled with adventure and happy memories?

Because I'd always dreamed of visiting New Zealand, I was ecstatic at the opportunity for a six-month work contract at the most southerly point of the southern island. Imagine getting paid great money to expand my career and travel at the same time. I was elated! They sweetened the pot further with two return airfares for myself and Marc, a "flat" to live in, and three weeks' paid vacation.

Married for only a year, Marc and I headed out. For the first two weeks we traveled the southern island in a six-berth camper van, taking time to explore the beautiful, diverse little country. Each night we camped somewhere new – an ocean beach, the base of a glacier mountain, or the mouth of a fiord. Truly, for me, this felt like a dream. The landscape of New Zealand was utterly pure, similar to Canada, but far more accessible due to its compact size. We'd be driving along the ocean watching the rolling waves, and within an hour the highway would climb into the rainforest mountains with perilous, undulating roads and sheer drop precipices.

The locals were friendly, possibly even more so than Canadians. Possibly. One particular offer of a free private tour through the breathtaking Queen Charlotte Sounds, followed by a bounty of freshly farmed mussels, takes a special place in my heart. If more people could try mussels while they're still dripping fresh from the sea, I suspect there would be a shortage. *Yummy!* You can't forget the pasta and red wine, of course.

A picture of New Zealand wouldn't be complete without the infamous and iconic sheep: sheep-manicured golf courses and backyards (watch your step), as well as sheep crossings on the main country roads, which could hold up your journey by a solid twenty minutes, depending on the size of the flock. I don't think I could ever tire of watching the ingenious, whistle-obeying border collies slink up behind stray sheep, starting and stopping by a tweet of the shepherd's whistle. I adored this country.

After exploring the beauties of the south island, it was time to get down to business. I was clever enough to find an employment opportunity for Marc to consider while we were there. He had an interview set up, and I felt secure Marc would be staying with me for the duration of my six-month contract. But something unexpected happened before I was to begin work, and I sensed the pull Marc felt to go back home. His Canadian employer offered him a promotion he felt he couldn't refuse. At the time it seemed like the right thing to do.

Promotion aside, this was an experience I desperately wanted. This country was my dream. I think, deep down, Marc sensed that if he stayed with me we would both fall in love with the beauty of New Zealand and not return home. Marc could never do that to his close-knit family, the polar opposite of mine. The thought of living abroad had lots of appeal to me, I must say.

After a sorrowful goodbye, Marc returned to Canada and I stayed in New Zealand to take advantage of my exciting work opportunity. Both our jobs took priority over all else, a common occurrence when you're young.

~~~~
~~~~

Sipping my tea, I pulled out an old, hand-printed, faxed letter I'd sent to several family members. This was in the 1990s, before we used e-mail.

Although I frequently expressed how much I missed Marc, I also had the most self-realizing, personal growth experience of my life in New Zealand. I was no longer absorbed in the complications of relationships or bound by any preconceived notion of who I should be. I was just me – Julie, with no past defining the perception of me. Here was an excellent opportunity to discover who *me* really was, not who I should be to fit all the labels that had begun clinging to me.

The sense of freedom I felt while traveling in this foreign land was intoxicating. Who knew I had such an adventuresome spirit? Who knew I didn't need to rely on the love I received from others to feel safe and complete? I missed Marc desperately, but I was equally delighted by how much I enjoyed learning about myself – not Julie the daughter, or sister, or wife. Just Julie, the Canadian. I loved it!

I felt empowered, strong, vibrant, and appreciative. I had many wonderful adventures, like the time I climbed Mt. Roy just after midnight on New Year's Eve. I headed into the night with two work companions, and we scaled the mountain's peak. With no predatory animals to worry about, our trek was a peaceful, invigorating, star-lit climb. Our ultimate goal was to reach the summit just before sunrise, making us the first people in the world to see the sun come up on the opening day of the New Year. It was exhilarating – that is, until I realized in the light of the morning sun that I was afraid of heights, sending me scrambling to a less treacherous section of the mountain.

The following letter, sent just before Easter, makes me smile as I describe my latest adventure almost two years before Marc and I started our family:

~ ~ ~ ~

...Things are plodding along over here. It's now officially fall, as we ended daylight savings time on Saturday. The weather has suddenly grown cooler and people are gearing up for winter.

I'm recovering from a nasty cold, but the cause of it was one of my most amazing adventures yet. I'm excited to tell you all about it! I was invited to tramp the Milford Sound Track in Fiordland, which is among the most rugged, wet, untouched landscapes in the world. I felt much more prepared for this tramp than when I did the Kepler Mountains after Christmas. I've been doing a lot of swimming lately, so I feel physically stronger. By the way, I changed my mind on the springboard diving lessons and may take snorkeling lessons instead.

Five of us went: my boss and his wife (David and Clair) and their friends, Donald and Sharon (also married with two young children). Sharon is a nurse where I work, so I see her often, and Donald is an auto mechanic who helped me to buy my little car. All four of these people have been especially good friends, and although they know how much I want to get back to Marc, they constantly joke about ways of getting me to stay.

Friday was a perfect sunny day. We did a little sightseeing in TeAnu until the bus came to pick us up and bring us to the boat launch in Milford. From the Milford dock we had a two-hour journey into the depths of Fiordland, the only way to reach this wonderful wilderness. The waters were ice cold, formed from glaciers, which in poor weather can be very unforgiving. But on this day, the sun was hot, the lake calm, so I sat out on the nose of the ferry and breathed in the beauty, thinking in quiet reflection and wishing that Marc was along to share it with me.

How spectacular the forces must have been so long ago to have heaved up the earth, creating those enormous rock formations. How magical for New Zealand to have been so segregated from other landmasses that birds could evolve without the need for wings.

Only thirty-six people were permitted on the track each day, so as to ensure a place to sleep in the huts at night. Those of us on the ferry came from every corner of the world: Americans, British, Germans, Japanese, Australians, and my group of Kiwis with one Canadian ... me. We left the boat at the beginning of the track, put our heavy packs on our backs, and were no longer individuals from different countries, but a united group setting out to conquer the wilderness for four days, knowing that if something went wrong we would depend on each other for help.

Reaching the first hut took only a few hours. We had lots of time to relax and make dinner, and upon nightfall the hut warden spoke to the group with some facts on the region. He told us about a spot where we could see the famous glow worms (tiny worms that gather in large groups in cold dark places like caves, sparkling like thousands of stars on a clear night).

On my first morning as I chewed on a cereal bar, a large chunk of filling from my back molar decided to break off. Bummer. This made me think of how things were in the pioneer days when you didn't have the luxury of a dentist.

On our second day the weather was perfect, but I started to feel a cold lurking in my sinuses. Great. I ignored it and forged ahead. On our third day the rain began, and it didn't take long for the rivers and streams to swell. Since much of our track went along streambeds, it was impossible to keep our feet dry. In fact, we were often up to our knees in water. As long as we kept walking our feet would stay warm, but after a full ten hours of physical exertion (today was the day to reach the highest peak of the trail) and wet-to-the-bone conditions, my lovely cold had taken a strong foothold come bedtime. Still, I ignored it, as there were more interesting and spectacular things to experience on this day.

Had it not rained – which it does three hundred days in the year here – we would have missed thousands of breathtaking cascading waterfalls that burst out of each corner of every cliff. Their beauty made all the wet moments worthwhile. It's almost as if you don't notice the rain anymore and become one with your surroundings. I rather enjoyed splashing through the streams and feeling the spray of enormous waterfalls over my face.

I survived to Monday, day four. My calves were sore by then, my head was filled with soggy cotton balls, and I could feel every heartbeat in my broken tooth. My nose dripped as heavily as the rain, but amazingly enough, I didn't complain. I was enjoying myself far too much. I just put my head down and practically sprinted the final rugged eighteen kilometers over boulders and landslides. I knew if I stopped, I might never get going again.

We all made it to our final destination at Sand Fly Point to meet the boat, each with individual pain, from twisted ankles and inflamed knees to sheer exhaustion. As a group, the satisfaction of making it to the end put a smile on everyone's faces and a strong memory in all our hearts. There's just nothing like being in nature as it was meant to be, away from all the noise and fast-paced lives we all live.

The remainder of my week I spent recovering from my cold. I'm just beginning to walk and bend my knees at the same time, and I got my tooth fixed.

I'm starting to plan my trip home, which should bring me back in about eleven weeks. Have a great Easter! All my love, Julie.

~ ~ ~ ~

I put the letter down and pulled the warm mug tightly to my chest. Staring into the fire, I felt the glow of that trip in every cell of my body. That journey was the ultimate reminder of how glorious life could be, depending on where I chose to focus. Although I had a few glitches along the way – my tooth, the cold – I ignored the negatives because I was so entranced by the beauty around me. I felt alive and connected to everything: the trees, the water, and the people from all corners of the world, appreciating each moment of my adventure.

I could feel the energy of that vibrant young woman work its way back into my head, like getting a new brain with shiny, fresh circuits: an emotional tune up. And I was ready for more.

Chapter 11

The Good Witch

December 2006

SHE WAS COMING OVER after dinner: the Angel Lady. Strange. One minute I didn't even know such people existed, and now I had one coming to my house. Angel Lady was an acquaintance of Lisa, my massage therapist. I'll call her Glinda the Good Witch, or Linda for short. Linda had some kind of unique ability to communicate with angels and spirits, and she dabbled in something called energy healing facilitation.

The ins and outs of this were all Swahili to me, but Lisa relayed information my way at a steady pace these days. For a year Lisa and I had a casual relationship, mostly professional, but almost overnight she became my bridge to the other side.

When Lisa suggested I should become Linda's first official client, my initial Muggle reaction was to find an excuse to be busy for the next few years.

Then I thought about Will and how many times I'd wondered since he was a baby if he was seeing angels or spirits. I recalled all the nights he would talk to unseen friends from his crib. I also remembered the funny round bubble things that showed up in photos of him. (I've since learned these are called "orbs," another term for angels). Will's photographs showed not just one or two orbs, but many.

I thought back to a time when Will was only two and a half years old, six months before our ill-fated, crash-landing, vacation-gone-wrong. He was slower to speak than Emma and used short bursts of words to get his point across, especially that night. We were on an early evening walk to the beach, admiring the clear blue horizon. A brisk fall breeze drifted up over the lake, bringing our attention to a plane and the white chalky line it drew across the sky. I pointed up to it with excitement.

"*A i r p l a n e* – see, Will? It's an *a i r p l a n e*."

Will looked up inquisitively, shielding his eyes from the glare of the setting sun. Then he pointed his little finger up like mine and said, "Cwash ... Die!"

I paused for a moment, trying to decode his words.

"What's that, honey? I don't think I heard you."

"Cwash ... Die!" he repeated, proudly.

What happened to *airplane* or *birdie*, or a word I'd actually tried to teach him? How would he even know the words *crash* and *die*?

I remained quiet and thoughtful while we walked back up the steep road that approached our home. Still confused and curious as to where Will came up with the thought that a plane could crash and people would die, I broached the subject again during bath time while Will splashed in the tub.

"So, Willy," I said, grabbing one of his toy planes, "remember the airplane we saw?" I swooped the plane into the air as if it were flying.

"Cwash ... die," he cooed again.

Good grief, he was driving me crazy. Why was he saying this?

"Why do you think the plane will crash, sweetie?" I gently probed, not expecting his limited vocabulary to appease my curiosity.

"Cwash, boo wader..." Then he put his hands up to his throat and made like he couldn't breathe, as if he were going under the water, drowning. " Gluaaa, bluggg, gluuggg, cough, cough."

My eyes went wide. Somehow, my two-year-old was associating airplanes with crashing into blue water, causing death by drowning.

As far as I could recall, *Green Eggs and Ham* did not cover this material, nor did *Blue's Clues* or *Baby Einstein*. My investigations into Buddhist philosophies over the years immediately drew me to the conclusion that perhaps this was how he may have died in a previous life. No other explanation made sense to me.

I tried to get more details, but his answers became sketchy. Will was no longer interested in my interrogation.

I told several friends this story and many agreed that my "past life" theory was the most likely reason for his reaction. However, only six months later we had our *crash landing*. Could that have been the connection? Did he receive advance information from the invisible visitors who kept him company at night?

Maybe Will got physically sick in an effort to keep us off that plane. And, when all else failed, perhaps those orbs – dare I say *guardian angels* – did their thing and helped protect us when our plane hit the runway. I've never understood how the aircraft could sustain so much damage, and yet, everyone survived. Divine intervention was a possibility, wasn't it?

So now an Angel Lady was coming to my house. As strange as it seemed, my curiosity got the better of me. She'd be here at 7:00.

~ ~ ~ ~

Will was the first to hear the doorbell. He ran to open the door and was halfway back up the stairs when I passed him. He looked up at me, and with a completely normal voice announced, "The angel is here."

"No, Will, not the angel, the Angel *Lady,*" I corrected him.

He looked back at me with an *If you say so, but I know what I saw* look, and then ran off to play.

As I worked my way to the door, I made a firm decision to do my best to *just stay open* to whatever came my way tonight.

Standing at the entrance, I swear she appeared like a glowing beacon of comfort. She looked at me with perhaps the kindest brown eyes I'd ever seen. Although her face was young and beautiful, her hair was shimmering silver, the most striking shoulder-length, white hair you could imagine. Maybe Will actually did mean "angel" in the literal sense.

I guided Linda into our formal living room, furnished with a bulky leather couch, a loveseat, and an antique piano missing its front cover, exposing the glorious internal mechanisms. The large coffee table in the centre of the room would be our makeshift treatment table. The warm glow of flames in the fireplace drew attention to our bookshelves, creating a relaxed atmosphere.

Linda sat on the loveseat across from me and put a deck of angel cards on the table between us. She began to talk about her government job and plans to visit her mother when we were done – all normal, respectable topics. I felt my concerns about meeting this Angel Lady quickly melt away. Perhaps I'd been a bit hasty to worry. In fact, I suspect she was probably more concerned about me. Would I be some kind of desperate crackpot, looking to summon the spirits of my long-lost relatives in the hopes of magically healing my daughter in twenty-six minutes? As it turned out we were both normal, everyday professionals interested in something bigger than ourselves.

Linda took a moment to prepare her energy, and then asked me to lie on the table. Now she would work on my energy field, assessing my chakras for imbalances.

The word "chakra" in Sanskrit means "force centers" or whorls of energy emanating from a point on the physical body. The Chakra system is a concept and term originating from Hindu texts and used in Hindu practices. They're considered focal points for the reception and transmission of energies. The most well-known system in the West is that of seven chakras.

Apparently, my root chakra (at the base of my spine) was blocked. Root chakras, I now know, connect us to our sense of security, both financial and sexual. As little as I knew about chakras, it made sense that mine was blocked. I gave her the green light to try and clear it. Everything she did happened in the air above me (my energy field), and although I felt silly the whole time, I continued the mantra inside my head, *Just stay open ... just stay open.*

The session ended with an *angel card* reading. "This is how I connect to the angels," she informed me.

Stay open ... stay open!

We sat on the floor around the coffee table, and she reached for her beautiful angel cards. Each card displayed the glory of the angels who are apparently out there at all times, ready and willing to help us. She described Archangel Michael, the leader among archangels, whose chief function is to rid the earth of fear and then Archangel Raphael, the powerful healer.

The reading was short and to the point. She drew three cards and gave three interpretations:

1. **Career Change**: I would no longer work in the same career. I was going to use my life experiences now and apply them to a much larger purpose, my soul purpose. I was in transition.

Well, that was indeed happening, whether I wanted it to or not. I could no longer travel with the business I had built for myself, or go back to the hospital, which required call-in duty and dependability. Therefore, I would definitely need to create something new for myself, something flexible that left me available to my children. So far, so good.

2. **Creative Writing**: Writing would start to become important to me.

"Are you writing?" she asked.

That seemed off base. I was not a writer, other than the many hours I'd spent over the last year writing letters to receive government support programs and various assistance of one form or another for Emma. I was puzzled by this card.

3. **Nurture my Inner Child**: In order to obtain what I was seeking, I needed to learn how to nurture my inner child. As I spent more time with my children and nurtured them, I would accomplish this task. I could not move forward with my desire to heal my child (Emma), until I could heal my own inner child.

And so the seed was sown. I looked up at Linda with the urge to cry. I felt as though she'd reached into my private secret spaces and pulled out something I'd long been hiding. Linda's message was clear and I understood it completely. How would I be able to fix anything within Emma if something was broken inside of me? I needed to address this part of myself, the part that mostly felt like someone else's life. I had never fully taken ownership of my own experiences as a child, and now it appeared that perhaps I needed to, for Emma's sake.

I had only known Linda for an hour, and by the time she finished I felt as if we'd been friends for years. As she left, she turned to look at me.

"If you'd like, I could bring you to my teacher. She's excellent. Maybe she could help you."

I can't say I was *excited* by the prospect of dealing with my childhood, but if it meant eventually helping Emma, then this was the least I could do for my brave daughter. Besides, when you get an invitation from a real live Angel (or Good Witch), how can you say no?

Chapter 12

The Mighty Oz

March 2007

THE MEETING DIDN'T HAPPEN right away. Linda and I had to wait for the next class date, but by March I was committed to taking spiritual psychology – a course investigating spiritual philosophies – and another class on energy healing facilitation. Over the next six months, two weekends per month I would drive two hours from home to expand my consciousness.

With no initial idea of what I was getting myself into that first weekend, I packed a small bag and we hit the road in Linda's red Jetta Volkswagen. We would stay in her daughter Jill's modest apartment. They, along with Susan, one of Linda's other daughters, already had plans to attend the workshop and slumber-party it together. Although Jill's place was jammed with overnight guests, they generously found a spot for me.

As difficult as it was to leave home, I also desperately needed a break from being a pancreas. Marc knew this and was supportive of my new, strange interests and desire to make my escape, albeit disguised as a workshop.

Jill and Susan were independent, successful, attractive women in their twenties, and I was grateful they were tolerant of their mother bringing in a stray Muggle.

The smell of freshly baked dinner rolls flooded my senses upon entering the small, cozy apartment. A healthy appetite always seems to follow me on my travel adventures, and I was starved. Supper was ready, but I couldn't help feeling like a child when Linda's two girls eyed us both with the *You could have called to tell us you'd be late* look. Had we any idea they'd prepared a delicious chicken stew, we wouldn't have dallied shopping.

"We stopped at the mall first," Linda explained, as I tried to look innocent, hiding a Gap bag behind my back.

"No problem, Mom. It's great to see you," said Jill.

Introductions began and we took our seats around the table. I felt strange, taking off from my family and spending the weekend with people I barely knew. As these three women laughed and discussed their daily lives, I was entranced by the scene playing out before me – two sisters, sitting with their mother, accepting her, loving her, and delighting in their unbreakable bond.

My sister and I can barely talk to each other without a full-on emotional assault. One wrong move and out come the insults, the ranting, and drama. I would love to have this type of relationship with my sister, and I remain hopeful we may find a way some day. Nevertheless, for now I settle for being the person my sister loves to hate.

As for my mother, I've tried to maintain a relationship with her for most of my life, but once my children were born I could no longer justify the stress of our dealings. I don't have the strength to handle the insanity that follows my mother around. I can't expose my children to what I had experienced.

As I sat quietly eating my meal, absorbed by the loving energy exchanged so freely between them, I felt envious and awestruck. The workshop hadn't even begun and I was already grateful for the opportunity to be *here*, accepted by people I had only just met, and to see what a loving mother-daughter relationship could look like.

The following morning we began our fifteen-minute drive to Leila's home. What a welcome reprieve with only myself to get ready. I actually had free time when I didn't have to think about organizing children, blood sugars, and carbs.

As the car traveled along Leila's driveway, surrounded by the forest, a sense of calm and tranquility flowed through me. A mystical aura permeated the woods around her home, and I imagined tiny spirits playing among the swaying branches. We pulled up to Leila's lakefront property. I followed my new friends to the back door, which overlooked the thawing ice below, then entered the lower level of her home, perfectly designed for intimate gatherings.

Several women were already seated, talking casually with each other. Most seemed acquainted. I noticed a small Buddha in the corner and attractive Asian art hanging on the walls. I was still clueless about what I was actually doing here, but I felt peaceful.

As I scanned the cozy chairs and sofas for my spot to sit down, in walked my new teacher, Leila. The list of her "titles" was foreign but intriguing: metaphysical minister, Reiki master, creator of energy-healing facilitation, and teacher of countless other natural therapy modalities, including this workshop on spiritual psychology.

Leila was born off the east coast of Sumatra in Indonesia. I was expecting, I think, to see my notion of what spiritual teachers were supposed to look like, but she was no Yoda or robed monk – just a small, pleasant, unassuming woman of Chinese decent.

Fascinating spiritual discussions around the topic of reincarnation filled our day. We explored philosophies of what we do while in spirit form, and how we plan our next human experience. I was riveted by the contracts we supposedly set up with our parents before we get here. I learned how all the experiences we have throughout our lives, from birth, childhood, adolescence, and adulthood to old age and then death, are fundamental milestones that carry with them a particular energetic wiring established from the time we are children. This wiring is something we apparently choose in order to experience the lessons we need during each lifetime or incarnation.

Considering the type of information we covered, I found the material surprisingly academic, presented as reasonably as any college course I'd taken. My analytical brain was serenely happy. Moreover, the bonds that began to form within our small group of twelve made me excited to come back and learn further. This felt like eating chocolate: after taking one bite, I craved more.

We returned to Jill's home for the evening and ordered pizza, wasting no time slipping into our comfy clothes to further discuss what we'd learned. When the pizza arrived, so too did Jill's exceptionally buff boyfriend.

He was considerably older than Jill and physically took up a substantial amount of space in our small kitchen, but his presence was gentle and compassionate. Our evening seemed normal, considering our day – up until my last bite of extra cheese and pepperoni.

As I sat with my legs crossed on a round chair, Linda began explaining the special gift our large, handsome guest possessed. He was a life coach of sorts, able to receive intuitive guidance for clients to help them with particular challenges. He didn't actually receive messages from the great beyond; instead he'd hear a name that often opened a door to whatever his client needed to investigate.

I had just made it through an entire day of spirituality without any strange experiences and although I thoroughly enjoyed myself, I felt slightly disappointed that I hadn't felt any great clarity on how any of this would change my life, or Emma's life. We discussed childhood energetic patterns, but I had so few memories of my childhood that nothing clicked for me. The theories were interesting, but I hoped for something more profound. More immediate. An ah-ha moment.

At this point, let me say I have since learned that answers to my questions usually come when I least expect them. This Oz stuff only seems to reach me after I completely let down my resistance.

I proceeded to ask Mr. Muscles how it worked when he counseled a client. "You're just sitting there doing your personal coaching thing, and then what?" I asked.

"Well, sometimes a name will pop into my head. This doesn't happen only when I'm doing counseling; it can happen anywhere – in line at the grocery store, in a restaurant. I just get a name. As you can imagine, it isn't always appropriate to approach a perfect stranger and drop a name on them. But when this information comes to me, I feel I should do my best to pass it along." He then went on to say he feels a responsibility to share this gift when it appears.

"It's vital *not* to go into someone else's energetic space without their permission," he finished.

Hmm… I had little experience with intuitive people. This man was perhaps the last person I would expect to display this ability. I needed to remind myself to *…just stay open.*

As foreign as it appeared, his gift intrigued me. But my left-brained scientist requires touching, tasting, and feeling the proof before me.

Just then, Psychic Schwarzenegger looked up at me with a serious, yet uncertain look and said, "Like now. I'm getting a name."

"*Really?* Right now?" I squeaked. "Who is the name for?"

"You," he declared.

"Oh, that's so cool. Umm, what do I need to do? Give you permission to tell me the name, or something? You have permission if you need it." I was like a little kid about to receive a surprise present. This man knew nothing about me. We'd been in the same room together for about a half hour, and now he had a message for me from the Outer Zone. I was ready.

He looked at me as if to say, *You sure?*

"Let's do it," I said. "What's the name?"

He drew in a deep breath, paused for a brief moment, then announced, "Ann…"

"Ann?" I questioned.

"Yes, do you know anyone named Ann?" he inquired.

Well, this was tricky. I didn't want to hurt his feelings or be rude, but I didn't know *anyone* named Ann.

"The name Ann means nothing to you?" he asked.

"Well ... ummm ... my middle name is Ann, could that mean anything?"

"Is that it? Anyone else?"

I strained my brain and stumbled again.

"Uhhhh ... my sister's middle name is Ann."

"So both you and your sister have the middle name Ann?"

"Yes, I guess we do," I said, trying to discern what the unseen realm would find so important about a boring middle name my sister and I shared.

Then, ever so gently, after several more deep breaths, he asked, "So, do you think it would be a fair assessment to say the name Ann meant something very important to your mother?"

Have you ever heard the sounds fireworks make as they whistle through the air and then explode into a glorious spectacle of sound and color? Out of nowhere I was standing with my mouth wide open, straight in the path of the biggest fireworks display I had ever seen. Boom! A direct hit straight to my chest. Leila, earlier in the day, had addressed the importance of childhood experiences. As much as her theories seemed interesting, I didn't see the relevance of the lessons. So just to be sure I was getting the message, I evidently needed a little shock 'n awe to rattle me up and pry open that impenetrable door within my heart I'd kept locked for so many years.

With one clean slice, the name *Ann* carved through me, busting open the place inside my soul that was supposed to be shielded and invisible to the rest of the world. I sat there trembling, suddenly freezing from head to toe. I was completely exposed and raw – my reaction taking me entirely by surprise.

With moisture filling *his* eyes, he looked at me as though he felt everything that was raging through me.

"It's time to go there," he said. "It'll be okay. You're in a safe environment."

I desperately choked down what felt like complete terror. How could I embarrass myself in front of my new friends by breaking down into tears over a name? Over Ann!

I wrapped myself in a blanket and tried to compose myself and pretend I was all right. I really didn't want to go there, hoping beyond all hopes they would forget this whole thing ever happened and I could go back to my safe, painless, unconscious bliss.

That was not to be. Slowly, throughout the evening, I talked about some of the experiences I had with my mother, trying to downplay events in an effort to not entirely freak out my new friends. I didn't want them to regret inviting me.

The next morning while I took a shower in preparation for our second day of lessons, memories of my past with my mother began flashing through my mind. I finally had a private moment to let down my brave face, allowing the soothing warmth of the water to wash away my salty tears.

I remembered stories of my mother, naked, with a shotgun, chasing my dad down the street and my dad having to race inside and hide in the bathtub to shield himself.

Then came memories of my cat Boots when I was about five, and how comforting he was to me. Another memory flashed of the time I consoled my sister when Mom left us alone all night and, of course, the fire alarm in our apartment went off and I couldn't do a damn thing about it.

I jumped ahead to the times when I was a young adult and my mother would call *my* boyfriend's parents to tell them what a horrible person I was, or phone my job endlessly in an attempt to get me fired. I was drowning in intimate details I had gladly long ago forgotten; all those times I had no control and was at the mercy of my mother's urges.

Shaken, I managed to pull myself together enough to get dressed and join the rest of the girls. I slid into the back seat of the Jetta, ready to head off to Leila's. I really just wanted to spin around and go home.

We were making the turn off the highway when we were flashed by the lights of a police cruiser, poised at the off ramp in a spot check. I sat quietly in the backseat, absorbed in my own world. No problem, there was nothing for us to be concerned about. And then I looked down to check that my seatbelt was securely fastened, as it always is, and much to my *complete and total* surprise... NO seatbelt. I couldn't believe it! At the exact time I noticed, so did the police officer. Like a lion pouncing on a helpless, crippled gazelle, he was over to my side of the car, asking me for my license and lecturing me on the safety of seatbelts.

He then handed me a *one hundred dollar* ticket and sent us on our merry way.

"Why me? Why today! I really should have stayed home." *I didn't even know a passenger could get a ticket!*

My friends looked at me and smiled.

"Kiss your ticket, Julie. It's a message for you."

"Kiss my ticket?" I grumbled. "You've got to be kidding. I have something for that officer to kiss and it's not a ticket! Do I have some kind of bull's eye on my forehead? Kiss my ticket!"

"What message did the police officer give to you today?" my friends asked, grinning with wisdom I did not wish to acknowledge.

"That you shouldn't be riding in a car when you've left your brain somewhere else!"

"And?"

I took a deep breath and tried to see past my frustration. I really didn't want to be spiritually enlightened right now. I wanted to be angry. I wanted someone else to blame, even though I knew better. I knew the police officer was not out to get me. He was out to do his job, to ensure people were safe. Perhaps that was the only reason he came across our path. Because, in my distracted state, I forgot to put on my seatbelt, and he was there to watch my back, to keep *me* safe.

"Okay, okay, I'll kiss my ticket. But I still think you guys are on a thin line of crazy here."

When we arrived at Leila's house, my plan was to hide in the corner until I could get my butt home. *FYI to all my fellow Muggles: you can't hide from those spiritual folks – don't even bother trying!*

I was no more than two feet inside the door when one of my fellow workshop companions bee-lined over to me. She took both my hands in hers and looked deep into my eyes. She smiled at me, the kind of smile that starts in your eyes and then works its way down to your mouth.

"You have three guardians with you," she whispered.

You know the scene when the Lion in the *Wizard of Oz* has finally met the mystical wizard himself? He's so terrified he actually runs full speed down the corridor and crashes straight through a glass window. He was face to face with something so much bigger than himself, or so he thought, and it became too much for him to handle. That's how I felt. My feet were ready to make their escape. I was topped up with enough woo-woo for one day. I wasn't sure I could take anymore.

"They want me to tell you something," she continued. "They want you to know that you are *very* loved, and that they are here *with you*, and that *YOU ARE SAFE*!"

And with that, the rusty door around my heart cracked open even more, allowing a lonely, frightened little girl, who had been locked up inside for so many years, to take a peek outside.

Chapter 13

The Crystal Ball

May 2007

LEILA AND HER SPIRITUAL psychology classes provided a profound opportunity for me. They shed light on how I'd manifested patterns in my life – how we all do, with our health, careers, and self-esteem. I was determined to "fix" everything I could, starting with a little handy-woman work to track down the moments in which my specific wiring blueprint was created. Was it too much to hope I could learn to manage and even change my circuitry through awareness and sheer will?

Clearly I'd fallen into a negative pattern during the year leading up to Emma's diagnosis, and I had no idea why. Leila stressed the importance of looking deeply within one's self, like gazing into the crystal ball of my soul. Somehow this would be crucial if I wanted to help Emma with *her* healing.

To be a good student and complete my assigned homework, I would need to investigate my childhood with more veracity. But where to start? I had little recall of the first ten years of my life. I prayed that my unconscious, sensing my emerging courage, would release useful tidbits to the forefront of my mind. I hoped for the ability to move forward, to finally free myself from the invisible, but real, shackles of my past.

~ ~ ~ ~

Pieces from my earliest beginnings started making themselves known. No, not in the Big-Bang kind of beginning way, but rather from my humble entry into this world during *this* lifetime. That's as far back as I can go with any semblance of confidence.

Spiritual psychology theorizes we choose our path prior to coming into each incarnation here on earth. That includes the people we will experience in our lives and the dealings we'll have with them to facilitate our intended life lessons.

The implications of this are HUGE. This means we "choose" our parents, and in essence stack the deck toward having specific life experiences.

Good God, who would create such an insane system? It is insane, right? Or is it?

The old saying "*You can't choose your family*" is essentially flawed if this is true, for we would in fact "*choose our family*." Apparently it's courageous and perhaps even evolved to come into this life tackling dysfunction, disease, dishonesty, and the like with people we make contracts with before we get here. The tougher the lessons, the more potential our soul has for growth. Great, sounds like a blast.

Of course, many different belief systems exist, and I think that's a good thing. Being a fan of science, I lean toward scientific explanations that describe the universe and all its contents as being made of energy. This leads me to conclude that the essence of which we are is eternal, because energy cannot be created or destroyed; energy can only change form. Therefore, it seems logical that Leila and her theories of reincarnation and all it entails are plausible. When our bodies die, it makes sense that we continue on as conscious energy, until at some point of our choosing we can come back for another human adventure.

Armed with this new philosophy as a template, I needed to look bravely into my crystal ball, back to a warm summer's evening in July when I was born. There, nervous and curious, I evaluated my decision to choose *my* parents...

~ ~ ~ ~

My mother was a young, beautiful, blonde who was adopted as a baby. She hadn't remained close to any of her family, birth or adoptive. From the stories she shared with me, she struggled with anxiety as a young woman and was left to "get by" the best she could on her movie-star good looks and sense of humor. Her deep respect and love for animals and nature was the one quality I saw that remained pure in her life.

If I had to pick a core theme of my mother's existence, I would say it was her test to find love and acceptance in her life. I've heard this can be a common challenge for people separated from their birth mothers. With many volatile and unstable experiences, she was left living on the fringe of society, disconnected from her parents and siblings as well as her own children.

I've always believed my mom should have received medical help. My father once said she'd been diagnosed with schizophrenia. Despite my numerous offers of help, she was also very clever and managed to avoid any type of intervention.

To this day, my mother lives a life of isolation. She makes the occasional attempt to connect with me, but I don't let that craziness back into my life when it comes knocking. I'd rather hide in the back room with the lights out, pretending I'm not home. Strangely, I don't harbor any resentful feelings toward my mom, and I'm not sure I ever did. I was frightened and confused, but not spiteful. She's my mom and I love her for that fact alone. Now that I'm an adult, I can say I'm grateful for the efforts she made to try and parent us – a role she was never properly equipped to take on. I truly want only happiness for my mom, even though I know it breaks her heart to not have contact with her children. I just haven't yet found enough space inside me to maintain a stable relationship in *her* world.

As for my father, I went all out and chose a handsome and compassionate, hard-working visionary, who developed, created, and built entire communities for most of his life. As a child he had been sickly, taking on the ravages of polio. By the age of ten he'd lost his mother from a cancerous brain tumor. I think he, like my mother, would have to deal with the feelings of abandonment that unavoidably occur with the loss of a parent.

As an adult my father poured himself into his work and his relationships, perhaps looking to replace what was lost when his mother died. This likely set the stage for his four marriages.

For a soul intending to learn how to truly love and accept itself, this would be an ideal set up for *my* evolution. With both parents engaged in the struggle of growing up without their biological mothers, the die had been cast.

The relationship between my mother and father was exceptionally explosive and ended when I was one. During a visit with my father, after ten years of constant upheavals with our mom, my sister and I were coldly informed by our second stepmother that we would not be returning home to our mother. She had given us up!

Well, there you have it; the cycle had come around full circle, and we had been abandoned by dear old Mom. In looking at this situation with new eyes – eyes that saw us choosing our parents – I could now see this reality with amusing irony.

Back then, however, learning our mother had given us up felt devastating. How could a mother no longer want her children? As an adult, I can see walking away was a brave, even heroic choice. She was unfit to parent, and her leaving protected us. Too bad I couldn't see this as a child. I mostly thought I had done something terribly wrong.

As I shared these revelations with my workshop companions, they pointed out to me that I was doing incredibly well trusting the process and being open with these new women in my life. This gave me the incentive to connect even more dots.

Perhaps my experience of being given up shaped the female relationships that followed in my life: relationships that reproduced the feeling of being betrayed.

Could my generally bad history with women simply be a recurring frequency, handed down from my most pronounced female role model? Perhaps I actually *could* trust women if I could change the dials on my internal radio to a different channel.

Before heading home from one of my final weekend workshops, I booked a personal therapy session with Leila for the following week. I felt good about this new path I'd discovered. I contemplated everything I'd learned about myself over the past few months. I was a a good student, working hard to find my balance once again, because I knew this somehow held a key to helping Emma.

As I drove home through the rain, I felt an urge to take a different route – then to my right I saw two words on a sign: Animal Shelter.

Chapter 14

Back to Kansas

June 2007

MOJO SITS MOTIONLESS, GAZING into the aquarium with the patience of a monk, entranced by the angelfish swimming about in their one-by-two-foot universe. I wonder if they ever contemplate the meaning of their existence. Mojo rolls onto her back in front of these graceful silver, black, and white creatures, checking out how they look upside down, as she gently pushes her paw up to the glass to coax them to play. Do they have any idea how much she enjoys them?

A tiny ceramic log, their only log, sits in one corner. They can't explain how it got there. The log just appeared. And then there's the bell they hide in constantly, perfectly poised in the east corner so the early morning sun casts a gentle glow through the bell's jagged entrance. This is the only world they've ever known; the only world that, in their limited perspective, could exist.

The sun, the bell, the log – these things have always been there and likely always will. The fish have never been anywhere else or experienced anything different. If a new fish entered the tank one day and tried to tell them they were all just small, contained, beautiful exhibits for other advanced beings to gaze upon, what would they say? What could they say?

Do they know there *are* others gazing down upon them, enjoying them, and helping them?

~ ~ ~ ~

I arrived at Leila's home for the first time on my own. I had no expectations of what would happen. I was beginning to finally learn to ... *just stay open*. My mantra must have been working. I followed her to the tranquil therapy room and she motioned for me to get comfortable on the massage table. A pleasant smell of Nag Champa incense permeated the room, putting me at ease. I lay on the table facing up, and then followed her instructions. I closed my eyes, took deep cleansing breaths, and drifted into peacefulness. I'm not sure if Leila realized how sleep-deprived I usually was, with all of Emma's nighttime blood sugar checks. I was beginning to worry I'd accidentally fall asleep if I became too relaxed. That could be rude, not to mention a waste of everyone's time.

Then I heard the faint high-pitched chime of a triangle – a lovely sound that helped keep me present and awake.

"Deep breathe in and blow it all out," Leila said. She repeated this three times.

She began to work in the air above me, assessing my energy field, just as she'd taught Linda to do. I felt relaxed and comfortable, and after what seemed like a significant amount of time, I began to consider how my drive home would be. *What should I make for dinner? I'd love to pick up some of that incense she's burning; it's so lovely.*

"Deep breathe in and blow it all out."

What's with all this breathing business? I wonder if we're almost done. I think I feel much better already. Surely, she must be almost done?

I considered opening my eyes. I still felt askward doing this, but I knew it was best to keep my eyes closed, to just stay relaxed and *open.* Then something strange began to happen. I'm certain there must be a rational, scientific explanation, and when I know what that is I'll be sure and share it with you. But part of me knows better. Part of me realizes we humans may, in fact, be just like my angelfish in their aquarium. Quite likely there could be unseen, advanced beings looking down upon us, enjoying us, and helping us.

I began to feel a vibration in my fingers. The feeling is difficult to describe except to say it seemed almost electric and tingly. Not painful, but intense. I told Leila how my fingers were feeling, and she calmly reassured me this was a good thing. She was raising my vibration, the vibration in the room, to better connect with my guides and work on what needed healing.

The feeling began to move through my hands and up my forearms. *Holy crap, maybe I've had too much air with all this breathing. Stay open ... stay open...* Then I noticed I was almost holding my breath and Leila reminded me to breathe again, normally, slowly, and deeply.

I tried to relax, but I kept my eyes firmly shut. I was afraid if I opened them I might see something too intense. Then the weird stuff started – things I didn't even tell my family about until I decided to write this chapter. My fingers lifted into the air as though I was a puppet with strings attached. They rose off the bed – first my right, then my left, then my forearms, bending at the elbows. *Am I having a seizure?* I thought. But I couldn't be. *I felt okay*.

"Leila, what's up with my hands?" I kept my eyelids closed, clamped tight.

"Many are here to help you today. The room is full, Julie. Are you ready to get started?"

GET STARTED? I was rather hoping we were just about done. *Exactly who is in the room with us?*

I kept breathing, telling myself I was safe. Everything felt perfectly normal except for my floating, warm, tingly hands. Then a picture entered my mind: Karen was holding my right hand, smiling at me, reassuring me. On my left hand was Uncle George, giving me a wink and a comforting grin. *Was I making this up?* It didn't seem to matter. Their images helped me relax and focus on something other than my crazy hands.

Then my thoughts began to stray once more. I saw myself as a little girl, maybe five years old, sitting on the opposite side of my father's desk in his study. *Great! Here I go again. I'm supposed to be staying present and alert. Why does my mind always wander?*

Leila tells me she can see me as a little girl. "What's this memory about?" she asks.

I could have broken the moment to ask Leila how she read my mind. But with my hands still floating above me like hawks in the wind, I flew above logic and skepticism and got right to the point.

"It's me," I confirmed. "My dad is asking me who I want to live with, him or Mom."

"How is that making you feel?" she said.

"Sad, scared. I don't want to hurt his feelings, but Mom needs me. I don't know what to say to him. I just feel like crying."

"Why don't you cry?"

"I'm too scared. I don't want to be here, but he asks me again. Who do I want to live with? I have to answer. I have to tell him Mom needs me more than he does."

"Looking down at that little girl, Julie, what would you like to tell her right now? What do you think she needs so she can feel better?"

"She needs a hug, a long hug. She needs to hear she is loved and safe. She needs to feel loved and safe."

"Then hug her, Julie, and show her she is loved and safe."

And so I do that, objectively, as an outsider looking down at this little girl. Standing apart from her, I can do this easily. Who wouldn't comfort a little girl in need?

Then my mind wandered again. I was in our apartment with my mom. I was maybe six or eight, perhaps. I felt as though I had been sucked back in time, back to Kansas where everything began. I was looking out the balcony window into the cold, crisp winter sun. We lived about five stories up, so I had a great view of our street, cars going in and out of the parking garage, bundled up neighbors scurrying in and out of the triplex apartments. I don't know exactly why I was home, other than I was probably sick (that was common for me). I was anxiously waiting for my sister to come home from school. I'm quite certain she never knew how much I would look forward to having her around, how much I looked up to her, how important she was to me.

I saw her round the second apartment building, a cold winter wind blowing her hair. Mom called to me, "Do you see her yet, Julie?"

I didn't respond. It would not be good if Mom saw her. She had *too* many ear infections and Mom told her every day to be sure to wear her hat, and she's wasn't. *Why could't she just put her hat on?* Mom came into the living room to look over my shoulder. She saw her – no hat, red ears – and the volcano inside her began to build pressure. I could see it.

My sister entered the apartment, unaware of the series of events already set in motion. The yelling began immediately. I did my best to stay out of the way, but it was difficult.

They were in the kitchen. I peeked around the corner. Mom was so angry, she scared me. Then it happened, the look of complete terror on my sister's face as the knife came out and rested at her throat. My mother's words: "I gave you life, I can take it away."

All I could do was stand still, paralyzed with fear for my sister, fear of getting in the way of that knife. I felt completely helpless to stop what might happen – helpless to save my sister – helpless to stop my mother from being so angry. Most of all, I felt helpless to feel anything but scared and unsafe.

I don't know how long it all took. The yelling, the crying, the moment my mom finally decided to put down the knife and let my sister live another day. I wanted so badly to make everything better.

"What would you like to tell that little girl right now?" Leila inquires once again.

I struggle to take in another deep breath and choke down my tears.

The Nag Champa feels more like a place than a scent. A wave of peace flows through my heart as Leila gently takes hold of my suspended hands and places them across my chest.

"I would hold her and tell her it's not her fault. That she is loved, and she is safe."

I hear her step back and breathe in the energy that surrounds us both. Slowly, softly, she whispers:

"Then do that, Julie."

Chapter 15

A New Heart

I NEEDED THE TWO HOURS to ground myself as I drove home. I cherished this time for quiet reflection. I laughed aloud as I recapped the volume of details that surfaced in my session with Leila. Whether I'd spent thousands of dollars on psychoanalysis or the mere sixty with a Lightworker, I now had enough evidence to blame all my problems on my parents, especially my beautiful, broken mother. If my Muggle perspective held, blame certainly would be the thing to do.

Mom loved her children. I never questioned that. But love alone couldn't nullify her inadequacies. Somehow, I must have known that when I chose her.

The dots were connecting once again, revealing more of my life's master puzzle: helplessness, lack of safety, terror of circumstances beyond my control. The tsunami ... Karen's death ... the crash landing ... Emma's disease. Were my negative experiences during these events triggered by a deep-seated, cellular memory? Perhaps viewing the images of that vulnerable little boy in Thailand pushed some kind of replay button within me, causing me to see life through the lens of my childhood trauma, attracting more opportunities to feel this discomfort again and again.

My family always seemed to have its share of drama and struggles. For the most part, my sister's ride has been much bumpier than mine. Despite my efforts to help, I've always felt like that little girl in the kitchen, watching frozen and helpless as the next crisis played out in her life.

No wonder traveling to New Zealand brought such relief. In that pristine place I was a world away from painful memories and triggers.

Why the allure of parenting, anyway? What's the point? With one moment of Muggle madness you can hardwire your beloved children with their own self-destruct buttons. I could spend my entire life loving and nurturing my children to the best of my ability, but five minutes of insanity could mess them up for life. What a daunting proposition.

I mostly agree with the words Jack Canfield articulated in *The Secret* when talking about "bad stuff" that happens in our lives. "... it's in the past; leave it there and get on with your life." Up until the tsunami I lived my life mostly ignoring anything beyond last weekend. By and large, I believed (and still do) it's better not to dwell on bad energy.

But what happens if the negative frequencies you ignore begin to interfere with living a good life? What if they hold you back from your true potential, like a flying pack of evil monkeys circling overhead, threatening to pull you back to your worst fears, where the darkness of your past becomes an overwhelming vortex.

Moreover, what if we do *indeed* choose our parents? Are they merely fulfilling their obligations to us, providing the experiences we need to reach our truest potential? Then who's to blame? Alternatively and more accurately, who is ultimately responsible for our successes and failures?

Could it be as simple as looking in the mirror?

A sense of empowerment enveloped me as I saw more clearly that taking ownership of my life would free me. I wanted to know I could use *all* the experiences I've had to grow and prosper, never again to blame or suffer.

I finally saw how I couldn't hide from my past. That I wouldn't want to. After all, it was all part of making me. If I didn't want "it" to hold me back, I suspected this was the time to embrace my fears. What an amazing opportunity I'd been given to explore and shine a light of awareness on this shadowy side of myself. Imagine if I could move past my childhood insecurities and learn to be there for myself. How could that not translate to being a more nurturing parent to my kids?

In the peace of my van, I thanked my parents for doing an excellent job, for showing me what I most needed to learn. With this awareness, I saw I was now learning from my experiences, no longer being ruled by them.

My childhood set me up for interesting parental challenges – things I never knew could be so all consuming. I wondered if that was also my mother's experience. Without the guidance of a mother I found myself parenting by the seat of my pants, which did have certain benefits.

I'm definitely not the type of mom who follows a rulebook. Instead, I follow my heart, even when a rulebook would be more effective. Because of my own experiences I never wanted my children to feel hurt or unsafe, to cry themselves to sleep or feel the sense of abandonment that can come from daycare. I could never bring myself to let those things happen.

I realize now that I had been protecting (or overprotecting) my children from things I hadn't been protected from. Somehow I broke my hereditary mold and provided the opposite of what I'd received growing up. I suspect there could be a more desirable middle ground, but if my children chose me to be *their* mother, then they must have known the game, right? Perhaps they took the gamble that their mom would defy the odds of her upbringing and be there for *them* unconditionally; that I would walk to the ends of the earth to provide them with everything I didn't have, and surround them in bubble wrap whenever possible. That's quite a theory.

Sorting through these realizations, I was overcome with feelings of gratitude toward my children for giving me the privilege of being chosen as *their* mother.

How fascinating it is that I didn't address my issues from the past in a more traditional, scientific, or medical way, which would be a typical approach for someone like me.

But what is the traditional way to address our problems? Who is it out there in the outer zone who hears our pleas for help in our greatest hours of need? Is it the universal energy field? Angels? God? Perhaps God is *all* these things.

Who says God is always traditional? Maybe God is the face of Karen when I feel her presence by my side. Maybe God is what I feel when I pet the long, soft, black fur of Mojo and feel nothing but joy. Perhaps God is a reflection of all that *is*, expressing itself in form, ever growing, learning, and evolving.

Would my life change for the better now that I'd thrust the shadowy parts of myself into the light? Would I accept my experience as evidence that unseen beings exist and wish to help us become more aware of the secrets to the universe?

Yes. But this was only the beginning.

One Week After My Session with Leila

We were out for a swim at our local indoor pool where sunlight streamed into the windows and danced off the ripples of water, bouncing refracted light into every corner of the room. We splashed, jumped, and raced for over an hour. We were all together – Marc, myself, Emma and Will – a rare treat for us, with no time limit and not a care in the world.

I took a break from swimming and sat quietly by the pool's edge, suddenly drawn to all the other joyful families in this tranquil environment. I found it captivating how the light created almost a halo mist around every swimmer. I saw heat radiating from each body, similar to air rising off scorching pavement. Everything felt uniquely peaceful. Connected and happy, my mind was unusually quiet, with no distracting to-do lists scrolling through my thoughts.

A young family opened the door and entered the pool, dad first with an adorable baby boy in his arms, then mom and a sweet little girl with golden ringlets following close behind. She couldn't have been more than three years old. This lovely family enchanted me, bringing back memories of when my children were that young.

I observed their every move, every nuance. The young father headed down the steps of the shallow end with the newest family member in his arms, the infant sporting a blue bathing suit over the top of his bulky diaper. Mom, drawn to them by her maternal pull, followed her baby into the pool, seemingly forgetting about her keen toddler who was still following close behind, like a duckling in tow. *She knows her little girl is right behind her, doesn't she?*

I watched, expecting someone in the crowded shallow end to notice, but no one was looking. The pool was full of people. Surely someone nearby would notice this little girl following her mom down the stairs and into the water, which was definitely over her head.

Nobody.

I watched as she went under, hitting the final step, completely submersed. Mom and dad, cooing over the baby, had no clue. Everyone else was absorbed in their own enjoyment. And there I was at the other end of the pool, watching this little girl twitching and wiggling underneath the water, flailing her body to no avail.

For an instant, time froze. Then I was running. I jumped into the shallow end by the stairs and before my feet hit the bottom of the pool, my hands were around the little girl's body, grabbing on firmly and thrusting her high above my head into the air, my eyes fixed on her face.

The light bounced off her already bluish lips and water sprayed up around us. Her eyes were open wide. Then, with a huge gasp, she sucked in a deep, raspy gulp of air, filling her lungs.

Until her mom and dad heard the cry, they had no idea anything was wrong. Her dad looked at me and said, "Wow, a lifeguard!"

Wow a lifeguard! That's it. Not "Oh, my God! Thank you so much. We just took our eyes off her for a moment. We're so grateful."

I wanted to reply with, "Your little girl just about drowned two feet away from you, dumbasses!" Of course I'd never say something like that. These things happen. I wasn't beyond my own distraction.

"No, no. I just noticed she followed you straight into the water and went under."

And that was it; they took their weeping little girl from my arms and distracted her with a game to help her settle down. All I could do was return to my seat at the other end of the pool, completely overwhelmed by the fragile and absurd nature of life.

My family came over to me, curious.

"No big deal, everyone was okay," I said.

But it was a big deal to me. The image of her innocence and dependence was so profound, her eyes so big as she took in that gulp of air. I would relive this scene again and again over the next two days, discussing it with friends in an attempt to find meaning. They say everything happens for a reason, so where was the reason for this? Obviously not for the benefit of her parents. They didn't even blink.

Then the connection clicked for me like another piece of my puzzle or a new brick in my road. As I pulled that little girl to the surface I gave her a second chance at life. No one else knew she was in trouble. No one else could help her. Because – They – Didn't – Know.

My session with Leila had dredged up old, suppressed memories. But it also saved a little girl (me) from a suffocating tomb, leaving me free to take in the oxygen of new life. I was free for a second chance at being a child again. The rusty door to my chest was finally open wide, exposing a fresh new heart.

Now I needed to learn how to be a kid, for the first time – something my children had been trying to teach me every day.

This time around, that is.

Chapter 16

There's No Place like Home

August 2007

EMMA LOOKS OVER AT ME with at determined glare.

"The dishes can wait, Mom. You promised we'd play Scrabble today."

I do love a good game of Scrabble, but my first response is always to put off fun until I can relax "properly," whatever that means. Usually, it means after tidying up. I did promise, however.

If it were up to my children we'd live in messy chaos every day. All they want to do is play, laugh, and spend quality time with Mom and Dad (of which I'd never complain). Not too shabby really. So, why is it I can't let loose and unwind with them more often? Why do I keep my time for fun and frivolity tightly constrained until I have the more important matters, like drudgery and drama, under control? What, pray tell, is more important than being with our kids?

My VICs ("very important concerns") are always running tapes, like an annoying commercial jingle I can't shake. Lately, I've been doing better about putting my incessant "to do" list into perspective. I refuse to put them above bonding with my kids, which means the house is never clean enough. Welcome to the universal challenge of parenting.

I no longer feel the same throbbing ache for reprieve from my pancreas duties. Yes, I still need breaks from organ labor, and frankly, from parenting in general. But I've become more of a nester, a homebody. I loved my weekends spent away, meeting new spiritual friends and feeling accepted and understood by them. I'm beginning to find peace with my limited Muggle abilities, while at the same time feeling more connected to my wise, intuitive self and my band of fellow seekers. But each time I go away, I miss my family more and more, and can't wait to get back to my children and my life. It pleases me no end to say that my inner child wants to be home.

~ ~ ~ ~

The final weekend of courses with Leila started on a beautiful August day. On the way over I couldn't help thinking about the profound shifts, the undeniable progress, I'd made on this spiritual journey. But I had yet to discover the magic morsel of information that could help me find a cure for Emma.

Perhaps I'd discover it this weekend. This was going to be special. Leila's good friend and fellow teacher, a Lakota Elder and Shaman, was hosting a healing Sweat Lodge, an exotic concept I'd only read about. I'd always believed in the traditions of Native Indians and their interconnectedness to the land and the Spirit world. To me, the sacred nature of their ways was indisputable, and I was humbled to have this opportunity.

Emma and Will helped me prepare a special rock to bring with me as a contribution to the ancestors. We called the rock Bob. We washed Bob and rubbed sweet-smelling essential oils on his tough exterior. Emma and Will took turns bringing Bob everywhere – the beach, the park, and our dinner table. He was now an official family member.

We even tucked him into bed at night, wrapped in a little blue blanket next to Emma. I was convinced the sweat lodge ceremony could be our opportunity to learn the secret code to Emma's healing. Putting all the energy of our lives into Bob in an effort to communicate this intent to the ancestors seemed like the logical thing to do.

Significant rituals take place inside the Inepi – the home of the traditional sweat lodge, and the rules were meticulously explained to us upon arrival. I learned about sitting within a sacred circle and pouring cold water on heated stones and imagined our host sprinkling those stones with sacred herbs and grasses. I could almost smell the aromatic smoke wafting upward with our prayers, songs, and drumming, reverberating off the hide (or in this case, blanketed) walls to get the attention of the world beyond my view. Our host held up a large hawk feather and explained she would whoosh the smoke throughout the circle.

When I learned that once the ceremony gets underway everyone is expected to sit in reverence through silence, prayer, or meditation, I was glad I hadn't brought the kids. During the ceremony, chitchat, noise, or unnecessary activities were forbidden. The area between the altar and the fire is considered holy and must be respected. Women in the Moon Time (on their period) are not allowed within the sacred circle or lodge, since their power at that time is considered too great. Those participating in the Lodge Ceremony should be dressed modestly. For women, this usually means a simple cotton dress (moo moo) or shorts and a big T-shirt.

Other details included asking for permission to be accepted by the lodge leader. Only then could we enter the lodge on our knees, crawling clockwise to the next open space. With four rounds, the ceremony gets increasingly hotter and more intense. Participants may leave at any time for health or emotional reasons, but once you leave, there's no going back without permission.

The ceremony can last anywhere from an hour to four hours, as long as the Spirit directs. There is no time clock. During each round additional Grandfather stones are brought in. Between rounds, the door opens to allow for fresh, cool air. I wondered if this would be when the Spirits who'd been invited might enter.

Supposedly, the intense heat opens doorways to perception outside normal thinking. Odd or unusual colors, shooting lights, and sounds are often seen and heard. When we finally got inside, I'd be on the lookout.

The best way to beat the heat, they say, is to pray harder and get out of your head and into your heart, which helps make the space for visions and insights more possible. People might pray out loud, cry, wail, or do whatever helps their healing process.

After learning what to expect, my group of twelve fellow spiritual psychology students were eager to give it a go. The day was perfect, with clear skies and warm air. I put on a comfy cotton dress provided to me and headed up toward the smoke of the sacred fire.

Thoughts swirled in my head as I struggled to remain focused on my intent. I want insight to find a cure for Emma *...a cure for Emma ... a cure for Emma*. I made this my new mantra. I had no time for stray thoughts and was determined to rein in my mental chatter today.

I proudly handed Bob over to our host and lodge leader, explaining what my children and I had done to make Bob special. A look of concern crossed the Shaman's face, and she made the decision to consult with the ancestors on whether or not Bob could join the fire. She headed off into the woods, and when she returned, I was told Bob would remain by the sacred circle and then return home with me. We still have Bob to this day. In fact. I think he was *too* special. Either that, or those essential oils messed up his juju.

The long white hair of our Lakota Elder host was the last thing I would see once the flap of the Inepi closed. She then began pouring water onto the first round of red-hot stones, the Grandfathers. The ground was hard and I felt a small boulder invading my limited sitting space, perhaps a distant cousin of Bob? It was uncomfortable, but I did my best to ignore the pain in my left cheek. The Inepi was completely dark and my senses were heightened. The sizzle of steam rose from the smoldering stones, sending a rush of moist heat over my entire body.

It sure is hot... phew... I guess this is where the sweat part comes in.

Beads of it covered every inch of me and my hair was saturated.

Sure is dark. Cure for Emma ... cure for Emma.

My Muggle mind was relatively content so far. *Okay, worse-case scenario, I'll lose a pound of toxins with all this sweating.* But then it started, that spiritual woo-woo stuff. From the opposite side of the tent I heard a voice, but not from anyone I knew to be inside the Inepi. This was the voice of an old Native Indian woman speaking, or chanting, rather. Her words sounded like an ancient Native Indian language. Her song definitely wasn't coming from our host, who sat right next to me.

Then another voice started; the far corner had been infiltrated. The two women I knew sitting on that side of the lodge were sweet, unassuming, middle-aged ladies who, I'd bet my last dollar, couldn't be giving voice to this ancient-dialect. *These voices aren't from this century or even the last.* I opened my eyes as wide as possible and strained to see through the darkness. Even Jim Carrey couldn't pull off this vocal show. I desperately searched through the shadows in the direction of the chanting women, fully expecting to see their heads spinning around and their eyes glowing red, but I couldn't see anything. It was too bloody dark.

My back ached terribly; the rock poking me now felt like a sharp blade. How was I supposed to let go and get out of my head and into my heart with this painful reminder of my physicality? I so wanted to make contact with the mystical outer zone and have the good fortune to converse with my guides (all three of them, by last count). If only I could hear their words of wisdom, something to help heal Emma.

But all I felt was hot, sweaty, skin-crawling discomfort. And concern for the two chanting women who I worried might require an exorcism before returning home to their families.

I did my best to clear my thoughts. But I was so bad at this, so easily distracted. I now focused on the pain in my back. Since the plane crash it was always there, like a loud neighbor with whom you share a wall. My constant reminder was now apparently angry because it sent jolts of pain up and down my legs and into my arms. I couldn't stay focused and feared I'd be asked to leave. Suddenly, I couldn't even sit up, but there was no room to lie down.

I scanned my thoughts for something different to focus on, anything that could conceivably be a "sign" from my guides ... a phrase of wisdom. Even a single word from them like "Hi" would have worked for me. But I received nothing, utterly and totally nothing.

To the left of nothing was my grocery list. Eggs, lettuce, and rice noodles. To the right of nothing were visions of my kids and the imagined looks on their faces if they could see me right now. Then, to the back of nothing, came those words I had written a few months earlier after a weekend trip to an *I Can Do It* conference ... something about being *no one special, here to save the world*.

That was me, all right: *no one special*. No out-of-body experience or download of an ancient recipe for a tea into my brain that cures autoimmune diseases. Just random thoughts, pointless words, over and over again. *I'm no one special. I'm no one special.* Like a broken record.

Okay. All right. I see you there! I get it. I'm no one special, healing the world. Fine. If you don't want to talk to me, don't. I'll just focus on this rock jabbing me and call it a day. Everybody else here gets to be possessed by ancient spirits and God knows what else, and I get hot, sweaty, agony. So typical!

As I pulled my attention once again to my back and to the small boulder molding its way up into my liver, to the ongoing burden I'd been carrying since the plane fiasco, I – wait – I couldn't locate it! The pain was gone! No uncomfortable feelings at all, anywhere. In fact, for all I could tell I could have been sitting on a pillow considering how comfortable my back felt. I shifted my weight to try and tempt the pain to return, to call out to it. No reply. My back felt warm, comfortable, and happy.

The native elder spirits went silent, leaving their temporary hosts content. Thank God! No exorcisms on the agenda for today.

As the ceremony came to a close, I sat comfortably for the first time. Neither my back nor the heat were noticeable to me anymore. My mind became clear and peaceful as my breath slowed. We shared our experiences within our circle of friends, but I felt unusually quiet and reserved. All I wanted to do now was go home.

There truly is no place like home.

Part 3

Where thought goes ... Energy flows

Chapter 17

The Mystic

MY GOAL, ONCE I RETURNED home to my precious family, was to slow down my spiritual adventures. This was easier said than done. I'd opened Pandora's Box and as I sped down this new path, it took some dexterity to even think about pumping the brakes.

Over the past year since watching *The Secret*, not only had I learned about Feng Shui, energy healing, and spiritual psychology (including awareness of my long-suffering inner child), I also squeezed in a wee trip to Indianapolis where I learned a natural therapy technology called VoiceBio Analysis.

VoiceBio appealed to both my spiritual and scientific natures. Combining graphs, anatomy, physiology, pathology, and energy, this technique seemed tailor-made for my sensibilities. I put it through rigorous trials with my friends and family to confirm that a computer program could identify all the notes in a person's voice and, based on the amount of hits per note, identify energy balance in the different organ systems of the body. Sounds pretty out-there, right? But being a medical imaging technologist, I knew the frequency of tissues could be determined because everything in the universe is made of energy and can therefore be calculated as a frequency.

I'll admit I was ambivalent when Lisa initially introduced me to this tool, but I became an eager student when it accurately identified imbalances that corresponded to the conditions within my family. Low bowel energy for me; absent pancreas energy for Emma; minimal heart energy for my father-in-law, but with high energy in the arteries, indicating cardiovascular disease, and so on. I was won-over by this mysterious, non-invasive tool.

Although I intended to scale back on my other-worldly seeking and adventuring, word began to get out about the tools I'd been researching. Inquisitive family members, friends, and friends of friends began calling. I was even asked to offer my services at a holistic women's retreat, for money. *Yes,* cash! Money that could help our bills. Money that would make my new direction less threatening to Marc. Money that just might save our house, which we'd miraculously managed to hang onto via unexpected infusions of government assistance and tax credits. So, as much as I wanted to be home, I was equally excited about accepting my invitation to work at the retreat.

Curiously, one person who encouraged my new direction with supportive and keen interest, was Emma. She'd been paying close attention to my wanderings this past year, always asking questions and agreeable to try whatever new-fangled natural healing modality I dove into.

I was relieved that Emma didn't resist my efforts to find more balance for her diabetes. In fact, it was an interesting turn of events when she began insisting on accompanying me. That's when I was the one to resist. After one dramatic plea, however, I cautiously agreed to consider it. She couldn't attend this time because the retreat was only for adults, but perhaps the next. This was good enough for Emma; she was happy, knowing that when I considered something it meant a yes, eventually. Clever girl.

Women's Retreat ~ September 2007

I was fully booked to do VoiceBio's for the day except for one session before lunch, so I studied the list of other interesting therapy practitioners: ear candling, foot detox baths, reflexology, energy treatments, massage – all enticing. But a practitioner who read something called Akashic records captured my interest more than the others.

Huh? This sounded exotic. The Akashic Records are a sort of logbook of all our past life experiences, including our intended purpose for this present lifetime. Most people tend to have multiple past lives with the same life purpose, as it's rare to accomplish your purpose in only one lifetime. We often require numerous kicks-at-the-can, as it were, just to scratch the surface. My curious nature got the better of me, and as fate would have it I secured an appointment with her right before lunch. I was excited, once again, to dip my toes a little further into the waters of the spiritual world.

I sauntered through the woods in search of the mystic. This retreat was a summer camp where each practitioner had her own cabin.The day was sunny with a hint of cool autumn hanging in the air. I've always felt comforted in the fall; life seems to slow down as winter approaches, offering a welcome rest after our busy, fun-filled summers.

I found my way to her cabin and with quiet curiosity sat down in front of this petite, silver-haired grandmother I was meeting for the first time.

"What's your name and birth date, dear?" she asked, before closing her pale blue eyes to pull my records from the cosmic vault of Akashic files, somewhere up in the world beyond my view.

"Have you worked in a hospital?"

Ready for business, apparently, she wasted no time with probing small talk. Her years of experience at this trade were obvious. I made myself comfortable and braced for the ride.

"Ah, yes, I have," I answered.

"I see you in a hospital environment near a large piece of equipment, something like an x-ray machine," she said.

Well, then. She had my attention. I worked as an x-ray and ultrasound technologist for twelve years, so this was a hit straight out of the gate. I imagined a small chance she could do background checks on the clients who booked that morning, but as I'd spontaneously made this appointment, sleuthing seemed impossible. I was willing to give her the benefit of the doubt. Plus, I was a little less skeptical than I'd been a couple of years ago. Desensitized, you might say. Stranger things had happened to me on these quests.

"I see you in a hospital, but it doesn't make you happy. You're a healer; you have always been a healer, and that's why you first chose to go into a hospital career. You needed the credibility of being a properly trained medical person, but not necessarily a doctor this time around."

I sat quietly, trying not to reveal any clues that might help her pull information out of me. My scientific side would have to test her. *I'm not going to tell her yet that I've always toyed with the idea of becoming a doctor*.

"Your life purpose is under the umbrella of a healer, always has been, but I see you moving away from that environment during a transition period that will take two or three years. I see many different certificates and diplomas. Being credible is important to you, to your life purpose. But you will soon realize that you no longer need those pieces of paper to prove your credibility. You will be doing something totally different from what you do now."

So far, this was still rather generic. Interesting, but no goose-bump moments.

"You've always been a healer," she repeated. "Healing is in your vibration. I see you as a male doctor, probably in the 1800s. You have one of those black medical bags in your hand. You're an excellent doctor for the time in which you live. From a wealthy family, you had the opportunity to travel a lot and learn alternative styles of healing, but most of it was frowned upon back then. I see you're still like this man today. I see you can't walk into a room without noticing people's physical condition and overall health. If someone needs help, you're compelled to go over and offer assistance."

Wow. She nailed it. That was me from day one. I can tell much about a person's wellbeing just by observing them: sore backs, respiratory problems, insomnia, migraines. I've been known to creep people out with my astute observations. As a little girl I would pick up gum wrappers off the sidewalks for fear they were shivering from the cold. I'd bring them home to my warm cozy garbage can, trying to make them feel better. *I had this strange notion that everything was alive* back then and that somehow I could make a difference if I just cared.

I was curious to know more about this male doctor person.

"I see you with a patient for whom you cared deeply," she continued. "A little girl with dark curly hair. She's sick. You go to her home for weeks, trying to help her get well, but you cannot heal her. It was written in her record that she would have to transition over. But she got into your heart. When you walked that journey, you regretted that you couldn't help her. When you went back to the other side, you both agreed to have another lifetime together. She would not be your patient, though; she would be your child. You would work to heal her again, but in a different way. She would help you get it right this time. Do you have a daughter who now has an illness?"

Alrighty then. Here we go. I felt goose bumps, shivers, and a lump in my throat.

"Yes, I have a daughter with a disease."

"Well, she has come as your teacher. You will not help her as a doctor would; you will step out of the traditional medical ways. Your transition to discover this path was a traumatic one. It was a wakeup call for your soul. This needed to be difficult to trigger the change for you, to move you forward from the medical world to your true purpose. This is how you wrote the records for your life this time. You're on the right path. You could have dug in your heels and refused to move from that traumatic place, but you didn't. You're on track. Even though you don't feel like it half the time, you are exactly where you should be."

She looked at me for evidence she was talking about the right person.

I nodded my head in agreement. I could never put my finger on the reason I decided to travel down this road, except it felt as though I had no real choice. I couldn't properly explain why I had such an insatiable drive to find a way for Emma to get better when there was no obvious path. Why would a relatively smart, medically trained person like me stray so far to the edges in the hope of curing an *incurable* disease? The problem wasn't so much that we couldn't tolerate this life. We were managing quite well by now. But somewhere deep down, I felt as though I made some kind of deal with her, a promise. I had to keep my promise, to get it right this time. What this mystic lady had said so far couldn't have felt more right-on-the-money.

After a moment of confirmation, she continued:

"If you are willing to work to your fullest potential, then you will begin to write about what you've been through, which will help others. This is the gift you have come to this planet with, the gift you will leave behind. Self-doubt will be your biggest obstacle. Should you come to a block on your journey, know the obstacle is placed there by you. You're on a mission this time to make a difference. Your daughter will help you accomplish this goal. Trust your heart to tell you what to do on a soul level. You will be the instigator to help your daughter achieve her healing. You have chosen a greater purpose this time around."

At this point she began explaining the logistics. I was completely thrown again. Writing? What is she talking about, writing? How could I possibly have anything to write about that people would want to read? A haphazard "woe is me" journal entry here and there? Please! I tried to explain that I didn't get the writing part.

"It will reveal itself when the time is right. You will teach other people that they aren't victims, no matter how it looks. You've had to live through that, to be a victim of your own life so you can teach it to others. You can't teach something you haven't lived. There was an option for you to stay in the victim mode and become trapped, but it was your intention to move forward. You're on a mission, have I mentioned that? It's a mission. You WILL bring your gifts this time."

With that, our time was up. I reached out to gently shake her delicate hand, which turned into more of a hug. All at once, tears burst from my eyes. My emotional display did not surprise this mystic lady in the least.

She simply looked straight into my eyes and said, "You're going big this time. Just go with it honey."

I nodded and turned to the door, heading back into the woods toward my cabin. I looked around the forest at the falling leaves. Everything seemed sharper, more vivid. I didn't want to go back to my clients just yet. I had some processing to do. Somehow, this woman knew my deepest feelings and desires. Even more exciting, she told me I would succeed in accomplishing my goals.

I stared out at the wind-rippled lake, breathing in the possibility of what our family's life would be like with diabetes cured. I still had no idea how it would happen, but I was willing to keep my resistance down and my heart open while I waited for the next signpost in the road.

Not alone this time, but with Emma by my side.

Chapter 18

Falling Apples

December 2007

THIS IS MOJO'S FIRST CHRISTMAS. She turns one in February, so we're still enjoying her mischievous kitten antics, combined with glimpses of the mature cat she will soon become.

Emma and Will watch as she eyes our perfectly adorned Christmas tree, studying the glittery red and green ribbons, decorative fruits, and homemade decorations lovingly handcrafted by my children. We know she wants to trash the joint.

I have little hope of keeping the lower branch ornaments in place as she targets them during multiple stealth hit-and-run missions. Her preference for the bright red dangling apples has us mesmerized.

"Don't pick the apples off the tree, silly kitty!" Will scolds.

Emma lies on the floor next to the twinkling lights on the tree and strokes Mojo's silky fur. She stares at Mojo and all the colorful glowing orbs with a deep and thoughtful expression on her face, and then glances over to me.

"Mommy. I can see color coming off Mojo, just like the Christmas lights. Have you ever noticed that?"

I look up from the book I'm reading, *Adam Dream Healer*. The book is about a young man who can see people's energy fields (auras) and about his unique ability to heal illness through visualization. *Has she been reading over my shoulder at some point?*

I squint at Mojo beneath the tree and see how it could look as though she's glowing with color.

"Yes, honey, the lights do make her look like she's glowing, don't they?"

As Mojo pulls us all into her world – a world that always brings a sense of joy and well-being – I reflect upon our past few months and realize they've been particularly happy. Peaceful.

I've been taking a nearby reflexology course every Sunday since September with my newest spiritual teacher and mentor, Mary. I've grown better at creating learning opportunities that keep me closer to home. My wholehearted focus has been on our health, which includes my own. I've made special efforts to manage my days around the fact that I don't get a full night's worth of sleep. As long as I keep commitments low, I'm all right. But it's a balancing act.

Although my life is quieter of late, I'm still driven to keep learning. I feel as though I've only just begun taking a shovel to the hard ground above the deeply buried treasure of true wisdom. I keep pushing the metal down into the earth to scoop up more clues to better health, more peace, and less fear. Endless options are available, yet they only seem to reveal themselves once I'm ready.

One of the greatest treasures I've uncovered are improvements to our diet in the form of fresh organic fruit and veggies, probiotics for intestinal health, vitamins, juicing, and shakes. Compared to the previous couple of years, we now seem boring when it comes to drama, catastrophes, and illness.

Thanks to tips from Donna Gates' *Body Ecology Diet*, I now use kefir (a probiotic rich form of yogurt) and eat less sugar. My irritable bowel issues have been much improved, and Will's eczema is mostly gone. Overall, our immune systems are noticeably better. Although Emma is still diabetic, I find I can improve her blood sugars with reflexology and regular exercise, plus an alkaline, high-fiber diet and vitamins.

Unbelievably, we're getting used to the diabetic lifestyle, just as the doctors said we would. It's amazing how adaptable humans are to the most extreme environments. I suppose when you look at evolution and see that birds could have evolved from dinosaurs, it's clear that life has the most amazing ability to morph and carry on regardless.

I guess you could say Emma and I are adjusting to doing the work of her pancreas, about the same way one could get used to remembering to do all the other automatically necessary functions of life. Did you breathe? Check. Did your heart beat? Check. Did you bolus insulin? Check.

No doubt, I'd prefer to have Emma free from the burden of diabetes and I'm still eager for a cure, but let's just say that being a pancreas-stand-in is no longer kicking my ass. Emma's been conscientious and responsible about her blood sugars, for which I'm grateful. My newfound comfort zone was recently put to a decidedly uncomfortable test when yet another local teenage girl with type 1 diabetes died in her sleep. This was the second beautiful, talented child from our small town in just one year who was struck down by an unchecked nighttime blood sugar crisis.

But when I push those fears aside and stand determined to forever meet the nighttime needs of our daughter, our life feels mostly normal again. Mostly.

I even felt brave enough to book our first attempt at a family vacation since our ill-fated crash-landing nightmare. We're leaving after Boxing Day to Hilton Head Island, South Carolina. Not flying, mind you. I'm not *that* brave. The plan is to drive there – three travel days in both directions – then a full week's stay in Hilton Head. Since Marc spends so much time in South Carolina anyway, this will be a great new adventure for the kids and I.

Thankfully, I no longer feel like a crap magnet. Talks about selling our house are continually postponed as infusions of money from my new, unexpected career trickle in. We converted the front playroom of the house into a tranquil office, because it seems I've become a bit of a "wellness facilitator." I still haven't gotten used to taking money from clients, as this doesn't feel like work. Between you and me, the people who come for wellness guidance have as much to teach me as I do them. Everyone I meet provides a reflection of what I need to do myself: eat more plant-based foods, focus on the positive, keep my intestinal system healthy, get more exercise, etc.

I love my office space with its bamboo trees, essential oils, massage table, white shuttered windows, and warm blue carpet. It's a little sanctuary I call my own and share with my new friends. I'm beginning to completely surrender to and trust in the flow of the universe. Although it isn't my intention to create a new career for myself, I feel rewarded by being able to help others. Helping people is also about helping myself. If I can't take my own advice and lead by example, then I'm not worth the price of admission anyway.

Yes, I *have* learned a great deal. Yes, I *have* made many improvements in my health and in my life, but have I sorted *everything* out? Is that even possible?

I still suffer from lack of sleep and the solution to this problem eludes me, short of *a cure for Emma*. Even the brief, rare occurrence of a nap cannot make up for a full night of uninterrupted sleep. If only close friends and family members of pancreases could be more helpful to those of us playing this part, but everyone has their own challenges and burdens to bear. If you asked me, and you didn't, I'd say that if you are close to parents of diabetic children or any other health-challenged child for that matter, learn all you can, and then provide informed help.

The worst thing you can do is offer idle, potentially useless support, like: "Oh, I'll take the kids for a weekend; you don't need to worry. If something goes wrong, I can call my friend who's a doctor." Like installing screen doors on a submarine, this is not the least bit comforting. In fact, it's a tease. You're there, you're offering to help, but we know we can't take you up on this type of support in a million years. You might as well say, "Hey, I know absolutely nothing about flying this plane we're on, but my friend is a pilot, so I think I'll give it a try!"

If it's the right time and place, I advise you to take it upon yourself to learn about the disease your loved one is suffering as though you were the parent. That's a lot to ask I know, which is probably why I've found myself flying solo on this ride. But when it comes to my children, I'm not willing to flirt with risk. It's hard enough, even as an informed pancreas, to do a proper job.

I wish I had more support. Lack of knowledgeable helpmates has created a major secondary problem: finding alone time with Marc. Despite all the improvements we've made, we still haven't sorted out how to reconnect with each other. We can never go anywhere and just be a couple. I pretty much function on that fine line of sleep deprivation all the time. With Marc's job being all-consuming for him, we still haven't managed to find our way back to the marriage part of our marriage, shall I say.

We do manage to get by on a day-to-day basis, but it seems we've been emotionally separated by the stress of the past few years. On the other hand, I'm sure some of this is the normal evolution of a long-term committed relationship.

Either way, I obviously don't have everything sorted out, which makes me uneasy about providing advice to others. I feel a bit like an unripe apple on a tree that shouldn't be picked yet. Will I ever truly be ripe? I don't know. Maybe never being ripe is what makes us human. Maybe our admission of vulnerability can help others. I know today's lessons are the beginning of an endless journey of figuring things out. The more I learn, the more I realize I don't yet know. Perhaps that's where true wisdom lies.

~~~~

Mojo takes another run at the tree, dive-bombing two more apples as Emma and Will squeal with delight.
~~~~

I'm blessed with such a beautiful family. I adore my children, my home, our town, our friends, and Mojo. I have more to sort out, but I couldn't be more proud of the improvements we've made so far.

"Ten minutes, and then it's time to get ready for bed," I announce, picking up the pieces of Mojo's destruction.

I head to the kitchen to finish the supper clean up. I wonder what will be next for us. This upcoming trip to Hilton Head will change the dynamics of our lives again. I feel excitement mixed with a bit of apprehension, as we have yet to pull off a proper family vacation.

Swaying at the sink as I dry the last of the dishes, and humming to the song "Winter Wonderland," I breathe in the blessings that now surround me. Emma enters from the far side of the room across from the kitchen, a good twenty feet away. She's watching me moving back and forth, assessing me the same way I saw her assess Mojo under the Christmas tree.

My apologies in advance for what happens next, as there are no delicate way to say this. But, as I worked, minding my own business, I, ah, well... I passed some gas. Quietly and unobtrusively, mind you. And unbelievably – Emma *saw* it. Yes, that's right, Emma *saw* me toot! She didn't hear anything, because it was silent (and not "deadly," thank you very much). But she *saw* it. I know this to be true by what she said, and the fact that she was too far away with music playing, humming, and water running to have heard anything.

Emma squinted in my direction and declared, "Mommy, I was just watching the glow around *you* and then all of a sudden it poofed out the back just now. That was really pretty."

"You just saw a poof from my back?" I confirmed.

In the past I might have thought my honest-to-a-fault daughter was making this up, inspired perhaps by the glow of the Christmas tree. But not tonight. I looked at her with complete astonishment.

"Oh, my, Emma. I just tooted, honey. Do you think that's what you saw?"

"EEWWW! Yes! That's sooo grosss!" She went running in horror from the room, screaming for someone to save her.

I dropped to the floor, laughing so hard that snot flew from my nose and I almost wet myself! Oh, to be human.

And so begins the next leg of our journey...

Chapter 19

Dorothy and her Posse

January 2008

OUR POST-CHRISTMAS HILTON HEAD trip was a huge success, with not a single crisis. We would have made the Red Cross proud as we carried all the precautionary items one could possibly need for a blood sugar emergency: Tupperware bins of food, fruit, and juice; chilled insulin, pump supplies, medical alert information, and a glucagon injection kit; cell phone, back-up syringes in case the pump had a problem, batteries for the pump and meter, extra lancets and strips, food scale, carb factor sheet, emergency contact information for our endocrinologist and pump supply company; and, of course, the kids. Can't forget the kids!

Diabetes planning aside, the trip was truly delightful. Our condominium was exquisite. Each bedroom had a private whirlpool bath and terrace. We had a modern, vibrant, yellow and blue kitchen, and we were smack dab in the middle of lush, green, golfing paradise. Each morning we awakened to ocean breezes inviting us out to miles of sandy pleasure. We spent hours exploring the magnificent terrain, often rescuing translucent, mysterious jellyfish caught ashore after the tide retreated during the early hours of the dawn.

Truth is, we could have done nothing at all except sit in front of the TV, watching Mike Rowe's *Dirty Jobs* marathon on the

Discovery Channel, and it would have been a blast. We were finally, for the first time possibly *ever,* hanging out together as a family without any distractions. No cleaning or laundry, no business or family crisis calls. This was everything I always longed for in a family vacation.

On the one day it rained, we watched *Dirty Jobs*, laughing and cringing at the often poopy adventures Mike willingly takes on. The rest of the trip was filled with exploring Hilton Head's elegant charm and history, starting with the Harbour Town Lighthouse and its extensive view of the island. Then it was time for an adventurous boat ride in search of pods of wild dolphins. One particular dolphin swam straight up to our boat, turned on its side, and made eye contact with Emma and Will. Very exciting! We also had the pleasure of what seemed to be the best shopping deals in the world in an outlet mall with outrageous after-holiday sales. I swear it was as if they were giving clothes away.

Sadly, it was over far too soon. With recharged souls we headed back home with the memories of our first successful vacation. We did it! No drama, no hassles, no catastrophes. A little miracle for our foursome.

After settling back into our daily routines at home, I was eager to learn about auras. I began collecting more books, starting with Donna Eden's *Energy Medicine*. (A pioneer in the field of energy healing, Donna Eden has been teaching people for more than two decades to understand the body as an energy system and how to reclaim more balance using these principles, and I adore her work.) Next, I devoured the remaining Adam Dream Healer books. Then I dove a little deeper into the dynamics of energy itself with Albert Einstein's *Elegant Universe*, and Gregg Braden's, *The Divine Matrix*. Energy was now my obsession. I essentially drank books for breakfast, lunch, and dinner. I couldn't get enough.

Energy, auras, the universe itself: all of this seemed like the same topic to me. Perhaps because I *do* believe E equals MC^2. As I focused my attention on these topics, the universe itself seemed to mold itself to my inquiries, just as it had been doing since the moment I asked for help on that desperate day in my basement. I noticed now, with great frequency, how information would come into my life exactly when I needed it. I suppose I could have kept my eyes closed and ignored what lay before me. Lord knows I was once capable mind numbing oblivion. But I didn't think I could ever go back to that. I wanted my eyes wide open.

Opportunity presented itself once again when Marc's work lined up another occasion for us to go to South Carolina. We would stay in the same condo at Hilton Head, this trip taking us away from home for two and a half weeks over the March break. By sheer coincidence, Donna Eden, the author of *Energy Medicine*, just happened to be conducting a weeklong energy medicine workshop at the hotel next to where we were staying, at the exact time we were scheduled to be there. *Can you say synchronicity*?

Emma and I giggled aloud at these types of occurrences because they seemed to happen almost hourly – from little things, such as finding the perfect magical parking spot or song lyrics coinciding with the timing of a conversation, to big things, like vacationing next to Donna Eden. But that wasn't all. Adam Dream Healer was planning to come through Toronto the weekend following March break, the day after we needed to go to our endocrinologist appointment at the Hospital for Sick Children, placing us in Toronto at the same time. Then finally, the icing on the cake: the Hay House Publishing crew was coming through the week after that with a lineup of our favorite authors: Wayne Dyer being Emma's favorite (she loves his teachings on self-development), and mine, Gregg Braden (I'm riveted by how he bridges science and spirituality).

Who could have scripted a more incredible line-up of opportunities for us? I felt almost as if *we* were becoming magical. For every question or desire we had, the experts would appear.

March 2008

The van was packed and there sat Mojo in the best seat in the house, perched in her cat harness at the back window. Yes, we decided to bring her along on our second vacation in just three months, and the children couldn't have been more jazzed.

I felt like Dorothy, complete with my posse: Mojo our animal guide, Emma my courageous daughter, Will my compassionate son, and Marc, the brains of the operation. We couldn't lose. What a turnaround from where we were two short years ago.

The drive this time around was even easier than the first. We knew what to expect and where to stay and eat along the way. We headed to the same five-star timeshare condominium located on the beautiful Atlantic shores of Hilton Head Island. Along with our diabetes supplies, we also had tennis rackets, bathing suits, books, and golf clubs. We were ready to enjoy the beauty and tranquility of our new getaway.

Both Marc and I agreed this was a perfect spot for us to vacation. We could drive here, we didn't need to struggle with language barriers, the golfing was world class, and we were greeted by dolphins at the beach almost every day – much to Emma and Will's delight. The weather was perfect, not too humid or too hot during the winter months. The locals were friendly, too. We felt as if this was our second home. It was the exact dream vacation we'd written out over dinner a year ago, back when I was turning our house into one big vision board. I remembered how Marc's skeptical stink-eye stares bothered me. Well, seeing as how my dreaming, or visioning, had worked out so beautifully, I couldn't help but rub it in a little.

"Would you ever have guessed we'd be here again in just three months? Are you *on-board* now?"

Marc was still hesitant. "The money isn't necessarily pouring in yet," he said.

True, money wasn't pouring in, but thanks to my creative accumulations of travel reimbursements through Marc's work, borrowed timeshare weeks from my father, and thrifty budgeting, we *were* here. Again!

Shortly before leaving for Hilton Head I'd enquired about Donna Eden's workshop, curious to attend a day or two with Emma. A full seven days would definitely be too much for a nine-year-old. And at age six, Will would be lucky to pull off an afternoon. Upon discussions with Donna's assistant, we decided it would be best to only drop by for an autographed Aura DVD.

On day three of our March break, Emma and I sat quietly in the comfortable lounge chairs with Donna's assistant as we waited for Mrs. Eden to meet us on her way to dinner. Armed with our books, Emma and I planned the rest of our evening, while Marc and Will played mini-putt at the condo.

We knew we'd be giddy after our meeting, so we planned a simple night of heading off to the Piggly Wiggly to pick up crisp greens as a side to the fresh crab we had lined up for dinner. After that we would stroll down the long stretch of endless beach to search for more sharks' teeth, ending perhaps with a swim, bath, reading, then bed.

Bedtime was always eagerly filled with plenty of reading – a solid chapter of *The Golden Compass* for the kids, and when they were asleep *A New Earth* by Eckhart Tolle for me, followed by watching a download of Oprah's online classes of *A New Earth* on my laptop.

Donna approached from the elevators with her husband, wearing a cheerful, glowing smile, her curly blond hair bouncing around her shoulders. We stood anticipating an introduction by her assistant, when Donna glided towards us, her smiling eyes fixed on Emma. She stepped straight past her assistant and reached out to put her hand on Emma's shoulder.

"Hello sweetheart! Am I here to see you?"

Emma beamed with delight as the affection and attention from Donna poured over her. This was a new experience for me, almost as if I wasn't there.

Donna continued to stare at Emma. Well, not *at* her so much, but *around* her, as though mesmerized. Our five minutes with Donna turned into a half hour of conversation about Emma's journey with diabetes. All the while, Donna maintained that glazed and entertained expression as she watched what I suspect was Emma's aura.

"You are a special little girl, Emma; the energy around you is so beautiful."

Emma looked at her with a permanent smile.

"You have a wondrous spirit and an old soul. I hope I get the chance to know you. Perhaps you'd like to bring your mom and brother to my workshop tomorrow. It's my day to teach about auras. Would you like to be my guest for the day?"

Emma's head bounced up and down. "Can we go, Mom?"

"Of course, we can. Thank you very much!"

~ ~ ~ ~

The three of us arrived the next morning. Several hundred people were present, all adults except one other girl a little older than Emma. We sheepishly worked our way toward the front right side to several empty seats, feeling a bit awkward to enter the workshop at mid-point, free of charge no less. Everyone in the room was a serious energy practitioner and here we were, curious, playful seekers.

I came armed with snacks and Lego distractions. The young girl targeted her sights on us within seconds of entering and joined us for what would turn out to be half the day. She was there not as a participant, but because her mother had no choice but to bring her. Now on her fourth day, she was delighted to find another child to play with. The audience settled in and Donna attached her microphone. Time to begin the day with some dance moves. The children enjoyed the silly fun. So far, so good.

Then Donna explained we would be discussing chakras, auras, and colors, but first she wanted to introduce a special guest. She gestured for Emma to come up beside her on stage.

Emma's cheeks went four shades of red as all eyes in the room fell on her. Seeing Emma's shy reaction, Donna suggested she just stand up for a moment while she explained to the audience the colors she saw around Emma: indigo and rose. Indigo symbolizes intelligence and spiritual aptitude, psychic perception, and higher intuition. Those with an indigo aura have deep knowledge of spiritual truths and insights. As far as aura colors go, an indigo aura is one of the most well-known colors, with many authors having written books about indigo children and indigo consciousness. A rose aura is the color of healing and health, peace and love, which validated what I already knew beyond a shadow of a doubt: I had a deeply insightful, intuitive, loving child.

The lesson wrapped up and it was time to do practice sessions on the tables at the back of the room. Emma and Will went straight there, despite my desire to leave. I was worried this might be a bit too much for them. I don't know why, but after everything I'd been learning and participating in, I still felt awkward in this environment, still Muggle-like. Before I could talk anyone into leaving, Will and Emma were already at their chosen practice table, taking turns.

Well, just for a bit, I suppose. I was hesitant to distract any of the more dedicated participants.

Will was the one to start. Holding his hands a foot above Emma, who was lying on the table, he said, "Can you feel where my hands are now?"

"You're over my feet," Emma replied.

"Right!"

"How about now?" Will said.

"Ummm, my stomach?"

"Right again!"

At this point, lying down on the table looked like a great chance to sneak a cat nap, as our busy schedule had me tipping my delicate sleep-scales. For fun, I hopped up for my turn to see if I could feel where Emma and Will were holding their hands, eyes closed.

One of Donna's assistants came by and guided the children on how to draw figure eights above my body in the air, saying how this could help me feel better when I get tired. It certainly wasn't difficult to tell I *was* tired; the dark circles under my eyes were a dead giveaway.

I closed my eyes as Emma and Will followed instructions to draw figure eights in the air above me, when all at once, an intense and overpowering feeling coursed through my body, pushing up through my heart to the point that I actually gasped out loud and clutched my hands to my chest.

"Wow! That's intense! You really *can* feel the energy," I said, perhaps a little too loudly. "Oops, sorry. That caught me off guard."

I proceeded to get up and let Will have another turn to lie down, when from the left side of the room, a fit, serious, silver-haired woman made eye contact with me and began walking toward us.

Oh, oh. We've disturbed someone. I'll bet we're being too loud.

"Hello," she said. "I just had to come over to tell you something."

Crap. *Here we go. I'll apologize straight away. I knew we should have skipped this part!*

"I've done workshops like these for many years," she said. "And I've seen a lot of different things, but..."

But ... here it comes, shields up, brace yourself...

"...I have never seen something as beautiful in all my life as what I just witnessed between you and your children today. You've really made my week; thank you so much for coming."

Wow! I didn't see that one coming. *I could really get used to this.*

Chapter 20

Hot Air Balloon

Two Hours Later...

UP INTO THE AIR THE KITE ROSE, swiftly, silently, as the winds carried our thoughts into the salty breeze. As if floating away in a hot air balloon, my mind searched the landscape, the clear blue horizon leading my gaze out past the waves. The promise of our greatest dreams was all around. How peaceful it is to give way to your visions, how intoxicating to see the control we actually have within our own journey. I feel safe, trusting in this new mindset and surrendering to be one with everything. Ah, to let go, and just be.

What a glorious feeling to be energetically connected to all that surrounds me – the ocean, sky, and birds. I watch my children laugh and run along the water's edge as if they were one with the kite, one with the wind. I feel such a sense of completeness, so filled with the endless beauty life offers. How could I ever choose to lose this knowing, this peace?

I have studied academics all my life, but none of it compares to the thrill of *knowing* in my bones that I'm actively participating in and contributing to everything in my path. How glorious for my children to have the opportunities I never had – to shed the tentacles of labels and self-doubt, to find confidence and strength from within, knowing the unlimited potential they carry.

This bliss was a teaser of divine perfection, as I could no longer keep my eyes open. My body reminded me of my fragile Muggle existence, the not-so-perfect circumstances that still present themselves in the midst of joyful contentment. I put my head down on the blanket and stared into the bright sky.

If only I could pull this awareness into every aspect of my life, to see the purpose in sleep deprivation and loneliness. Yes, challenges continued to brew beneath the delicate umbrella of my family. If only I could take away some of Marc's work-related stress, perhaps that would translate into more closeness between us. If only I could take Emma's disease away and get a whole night of sleep again.

"Let's head back to the condo, guys," I called out. "If we don't leave soon I may fall asleep right here on the beach."

I dragged all our gear, pushing myself along with every step. *I wonder if the intensity of my exhaustion has anything to do with the energy work the kids did on me?*

"Who's up for a movie?" I asked, not exactly a question, as I extracted *Harry Potter* from his cover and fed it into the DVD player. Every inch of me was done, my brain literally turning OFF. With all the strength I had left, I sent an emergency email to Marc, asking him to pick up a pizza on his way back from work. I was crashing, hard.

My eyes closed as Hagrid flew his motorbike down from the sky to Harry's home on 4 Privet Drive. If only I could be truly magical, give myself a spell to stay awake, to cease needing sleep, for that matter. Marc must get so annoyed with my lack of stamina.

We had come a long way, to be sure. But we still had a long way to go. I needed to focus my thoughts correctly, not dwell on the negative. If I could send my intentions out for help in these remaining areas of struggle, surely the answers would reveal themselves. I now knew to ask the universe for support, and I trusted my ability to hear the answers. I had faith that all would be revealed when the time was right – when I was ready to receive.

~ ~ ~ ~

I woke up to the smell of pizza and a husband picking up the pieces of our day. The company to which he devoted himself was beginning to extract pieces of his soul; he had to take a working vacation because of his employers' needs. Fatal ownership errors placed his job in jeopardy, and the signs of worry marked his face. This vacation was occurring during a critical time for us, a time when we could use the joy of a quality family experience together to focus on the future, not the potential gloom and doom that lay ahead for the failing company to which he'd been a slave far too long.

What a perfect moment to construct new dreams – dreams of Daddy being more available to his wife and children and less chained to an employer who kept forgetting how important its employees were. If only Marc could find a career over which he had more control and through which he could contribute to the happiness of not only our family, but the planet as well. Perhaps this could be a company of his own, doing something beneficial with his expertise in wood and logistics. If we could create our lives, then why not create the perfect career?

I did my best to clear the sleep from my brain. Marc wanted to tell me about a friend who was getting into bio energy, perhaps an area worth investigating. Every dream has to start somewhere, and so another seed was sown during our drive back home from Hilton Head, with Marc contemplating the potential of ecologically clean, renewable fuel sources.

We returned home safely from this second wonderful trip, but our traveling wasn't over. The following weeks fulfilled our commitments to see more authors. Our experiences at these events were always similar, with Emma acting as the lightning rod for miraculous connections.

Adam Dream Healer was kind to Emma and offered visualization advice regarding the pancreas. Then, with six of my dearest spiritual friends, we attended my second Hay House "I Can Do It" conference. Hay House is a publishing company founded in 1987 that began with a powerful little book called, *You Can Heal Your Life* by Louise Hay, the highly respected queen of self-help. Countless inspirational new age and self-help authors come together to share their messages at these "I Can Do It" conferences, and people who meet there often become lifelong friends.

On our first night we listened to Dr. Wayne Dyer. I loved watching Emma hang on every word he spoke and how the adults around us would study every expression on Emma's face. How is it a nine-year-old girl could truly be interested in the words of a sophisticated, wise, self-help speaker? Nevertheless, she was.

When it came time to get our books signed, Emma was hoisted into the arms of the crowd at Dr. Dyer's request. After a short conversation with us both as to why Emma was there, he proceeded to plant a compassionate kiss on her cheek before whispering a personal message of inspiration in her ear, "Change your thoughts – change your disease!"

I looked at this little girl, brimming with so much wisdom. I marveled at how she could get the whole crowd engaged in her presence. Having Emma at these events was a bit like bringing a puppy into the schoolyard, or like a man holding a baby in the park. Emma was a magnet for spiritually enlightened teachers of all stripes, and a catalyst for bringing more insight into my own life.

By September, our whirlwind of author workshops ended with Emma's final request of the year: a trip back to Toronto to see Esther Hicks (an inspirational author and speaker on the Law of Attraction) on her tenth birthday. That was it. No special party, just a trip to see the author of her newest read, the *Sara* series.

Emma was the *only* child attending this workshop of perhaps a thousand people, and the only person permitted to go backstage afterward to meet Esther in person and get her books signed. Esther told Emma what a special, old soul she was.

An old soul: there it was again. I've known it from the day she was born. She is much older and wiser than me, which to be honest, adds a special challenge to parenting. I rarely get to use lines like, "Because I said so!" or "I told you so." At the end of the day, much to my chagrin, Emma's usually right. Providing the logical and reasonable answers her linear brain requires can feel like a full-time job.

In the back of my mind, although I remained hopeful these adventures would lead to Emma's cure, my desperation for the outcome no longer plagued me. Dozens of positive changes had come about since her diagnosis: our unique bond, improved health and outlook on life, and the knowledge of a much larger picture of our existence.

We ended 2008 with appreciation for all we had and embraced the first half of 2009 with visions of a possible new career for Marc. Will drew us into his exciting new pursuits of hockey and music, while Emma poured her energy into being an exceptional student, with the occasional discussion about colors she could see beaming from around certain people. These occurrences were infrequent and eventually disappeared as she grew a little older.

I did my best to balance our worlds while seeing the occasional client in my humble home office. I knew our lives would continue to change, but some things need time, and patience.

Chapter 21

Is it Just a Dream

July 2009

I'M IN A SHACK ON THE EDGE of the ocean. Low-lying clouds cover the night sky like a blanket of ink. I can feel an approaching storm in the warm, moist air. I know I should be somewhere safer than this jagged rock island a mile offshore. I'm not even sure what I'm doing in this flimsy structure at night, alone. I begin swimming through warm, salty water as dark as the sky. I don't want to know what might be lurking beneath my gliding body, so I swim with the agility of a dolphin. Moving too quickly for any predator to detect me, I need to return to shore before the storm hits.

Then, as quickly as I entered the water, I find myself pulled onto land, dry and focused. My thoughts shift into high gear. Many people are out walking tonight; I must warn them of the coming danger. I need to find my family and get them to safety. Just as I have that thought, Marc is behind me, pointing down the shoreline, assuring me our children are safe and motioning for me to follow him. We begin the journey down the beach, telling everyone to move to higher ground. I look over my left shoulder into the ominous blend of black water and sky and see a massive, threatening wall, slowly building. Water on the shoreline begins to recede, pulling into the deep and exposing the ocean floor. The torrent of water expands and groans.

With instant communication through a mere glance, Marc and I pull right into the trees, heading for safer terrain. Our sole focus is to escape the huge wave rolling toward shore with the sound of a jet engine.

I feel strong, not at all afraid. I know I can run faster than any wave. I feel a surge of energy coursing through my body as we come upon a city all lit up and bustling with activity, sparkling in the night like a city of emeralds.

"I need to take you somewhere," Marc says. But he no longer looks like Marc. He's just some man guiding me into an office building. I believe it's a doctor's office, where a group of people are waiting for me.

"What's this all about?" I ask the gathered strangers, who look at me with concern. "Why am I here?"

"You know why," they say at once, eyes fixed on me.

"Is this about diabetes?" I ask, confused.

"You know what it's about." Their voices are ice cold.

They're staring, trying to read my thoughts before I even know what they are. For a moment I feel the strength begin to seep out of me, pulling into the direction of their stares. Then I take a deep breath, so deep I threaten to suck every bit of oxygen from the room.

"Oh, you mean the other thing?" I smirk, as my power rushes back into my body with awareness so sharp I can hear and feel the pulse of every person in the room.

Their eyes widen as they realize I'm no longer afraid of them. No longer afraid of my secret ... no longer interested in covering up the truth.

"This thing?" I lay my hands out toward the table with complete ease. Energy pours through my hands and lifts the table into the air, sending the group of concerned interrogators scrambling to the four corners of the room.

I turn for the door, hearing the buzz of nervous chatter behind me. They have no power over me anymore. Today, I choose not to be afraid. Today, I will show them just how strong and powerful I am. I don't care who knows anymore. There may be many out there who don't approve, but that no longer affects me.

I make it to the front door of the glittery glass office building and put my hands out again as I send energy to open the doors. Spectators are now gathering, both curious and unsure what to make of the glowing woman with a magical force they've never seen.

I stand on the sidewalk. The dark night has turned into a clear, sunny day. A fresh breeze heralds a new start for me. I no longer feel lost and unsure. I made it back to my invincible self, stronger than ever. I don't care who's watching me as I gaze at the awestruck crowd. I take in another deep breath, close my eyes, and spring into the air with the speed and stealth of an eagle.

I glide straight up into the heavens above the shimmering emerald city, soaring through the air with the greatest of ease. This is me, the real me, the person I will never deny again. I feel happy and free and gloriously alive.

~ ~ ~ ~

I sense the vibe of a stare again, a pull that immediately yanks me into wakefulness. This time it's Emma, pointing to the clock: 9:30 a.m.

"Are you going to sleep all day?"

"Wow, it's late!" I look over at my new shades, no longer the broken blinds the sun used to explode through each morning. Our bedroom is more cave-like now, more conducive to sleeping-in.

"Guess we should get some breakfast," I say. "I just had the greatest dream."

~ ~ ~ ~

By early afternoon I begin packing for my trip. Mojo leaps in and out of my bags, playing hide-and-seek. I come up from the basement with baskets of laundry and she goes bonkers, chasing renegade socks and diving under piles of folded clothes. She leaps to the top of the stairs with her back all curved up and her tail puffed out like a broom.

"Yes, I see you. Very scary!"

I have a hunch she's excited for me somehow. She knows something's up as I check over my "things to pack" list, deliberately trying not to overdo. I've been content and happy lately, but it seems I've hit a plateau. Marc and I aren't making any progress within our relationship, and I'm beginning to wonder if we both might die of solitude should it go on much longer. Deep down I know something needs to shift, and soon. I've tried everything I can think of to approach the lack of connection between us, but to no avail.

Finally, last week in frustration, I released my anxiety over the matter. Perhaps, all my concerns for our "problem" were only serving to provide that dreaded resistance to finding a solution. There is a solution out there, as Dr. Wayne Dyer says. *There's a solution to every problem.* I just need to stay open to it... *Just stay open.*

Quite spontaneously, I became overwhelmingly convinced I needed to have a break on my own – an entire week to sleep through every night, a vacation from my pancreas duties, a chance to evaluate where I am and where I want to go. Of course the only way to do that is to go somewhere on my own, because Marc is the only other person who can tend to Emma's needs.

I set my sights on another "I Can Do It" event. I knew I would enjoy it completely, and this one happened to be a writer's workshop on a cruise to Alaska. I still wasn't overly thrilled by the whole idea of becoming a writer, but I *had* secretly been journaling thoughts and events since the concept was suggested to me. Maybe I could learn to organize what I'd been scribbling about into something more ambitious.

I gathered all my courage to explain to Marc my impulsive (and perhaps selfish) plan to go away for over a week, softening the blow by accepting some part-time shifts doing ultrasound at the hospital to cover the costs. Then I confessed the part about the writer's workshop.

"Since when are you a writer?" Marc asked.

Let's just say my reaction wasn't pretty. At forty years of age, I had paid my dues as a mother – as a pancreas! With tears flying in every direction, I explained how I had to go. Maybe I would learn a little something about writing along the way, but regardless, I simply had to do this.

The timing was awkward. Our dear friends had just separated, and we'd been dragged into the center of their horrible mess. Every day was traumatic, with crying phone calls and urgent text messages. Matters were becoming more complicated as I noticed the wife in this equation, one of my girlfriends, seemed to be finding less comfort in my support and more in Marc's.

Watching how much she was leaning on my man felt a bit disconcerting. I could see the connection between them growing with each of her frequent visits for consolation. Even Emma approached me in the kitchen one afternoon after watching them engrossed in conversation by the pool.

"Mommy, she's single now, but Daddy isn't. This isn't right. You should stop them." Her genuine concern touched and worried me.

"Oh, no, honey, we're all close friends," I said. "I'm not worried about something like that." I tried to convince both of us. *I'm an enlightened person now; no longer a crap magnet,* I told myself. I trusted my husband and loved them both and was not going to let my imagination get the better of me.

While part of me wanted to stay and defend my territory like a wolf defending her pups, a larger part of me wanted to escape on this trip and hide from what I saw clearly happening before my eyes.

I managed to muster my courage and explain my concerns to Marc. He didn't deny the situation, only promised nothing would happen while I was away. I could have asked her not to visit in my absence, but I saw that as a means to push them closer together. Nothing could possibly happen – right?

With Mojo hot on my heels, I zipped the last of my bags and brought them downstairs. I lifted her up and buried my face in her soft fur, breathing in her happy smell. Will said goodbye easily, as he didn't really understand how long I'd be away. Emma clung to me like a spider monkey, desperately pleading for me to bring her along.

"How can you possibly meet Louise Hay without me?" she said.

A fair question. But this was a trip I had to take alone. After a zillion hugs and goodbye kisses, I wrapped up my teary farewell by looking around my home, the strength of my dream filling my body as I put my bags in the car. *I can do this. I must do this, for me!* I gave Emma and Will one final hug, and then made the effort to hug Marc, a gesture he barely returned.

As I got into the car, I glanced back at my husband for what suddenly felt like the last time. A strange numbness came over me. *Who am I kidding that nothing will happen?* Somewhere, deep down I knew this was a defining moment for us, and yet I had to leave. I would trust my overpowering gut instinct this time, even though it didn't make any sense. I needed to let this thing run its course. I had faith in my instincts to walk away, regardless of the outcome.

Although I knew things were going to be different, I headed off to the airport, unaware of the many details that lay ahead for us. Apparently, it was time for more change. Change I'd no doubt prayed for.

Chapter 22

Wake-up Call

July 2009

ONCE I LEFT, IT TOOK ME THREE days to stop counting carbs, obsessing about insulin, and realize I wasn't the diabetic. God, I needed this break!

My assigned roommate on the ship was an enterprising, joyous angel of a person, a perfect companion for me. While I had fantasized about sleeping – oh glorious sleeping – she had already met half the people on the ship and pulled me into the voyage with both feet. Before I had anything to say about it, I began having a wonderful time, despite missing my family and being uncertain about the fate of my marriage.

Hundreds of people from around the world had gathered on the MS Amsterdam. We were a united group of spiritual seekers looking to experience the wonders of our beautiful planet.

The writing workshops were motivating and encouraging, while also grounded in outlining the hard work ahead of us. I met incredible people who didn't question my talent, but inspired me to try my hand at this curious new obsession.

I finally had the time I needed to look deeply at the dynamics of my life, to step out of my self-contained aquarium and view the situation at home with a fresh perspective. I could feel my new frequency forming, one that felt confident in my future and what I wanted. No more gray lines for me. This was a time for happiness in all areas of my life.

As the cruise drew to a close, I worked my way up to the bow of the ship, to its very peak. The wind blew my hair off my face, and I felt a strong sense of déjà vu. I remembered sitting on my living room floor two years earlier, going through the New Zealand albums. Here I was, alone once again, experiencing another such rebirth. Gliding atop glacier waters on a boat filled with multinational friends, I felt strong and alive. Maybe it was just the fact that I'd slept through each night for a week and eaten the most incredible food. Whatever it was, I knew that I could handle my next steps.

I missed my children so much I could smell the shampoo in Emma and Will's hair, but the freedom from distraction was a lifesaver. At last I had the opportunity to clearly see my actual accomplishments and contributions, and the undeniable, unwavering, indisputable truth that MY THOUGHTS DO CREATE MY LIFE. I am a walking, talking transistor radio sending out my feelings, desires, and fears – a radio that doubles as a magnet; a powerful, never failing magnet that pulls me toward my next experience, or to be more precise, my quantum possibility.

I wasn't sure what awaited me at home, but I was excited about a future in which I was an active participant. I could view this future with an open mind and take responsibility for it – a future I knew, on some level, affected the lives of everyone else on this planet.

And yet, as I admired the majestic Alaskan waters, marveling at the breathtaking forces that created this glorious globe, I couldn't help feeling anxiety sneak back into my Muggle mind. Things would get worse before they got better. I knew that for certain. Now it was time to go home and face my future.

August 2009

What do you do when the love of your life no longer looks at you with desire? What if you can't even remember those blissful, soul mate moments of finishing one another's sentences, sharing the last bite of a decadent dessert, and reaching out for each other everywhere?

Is it possible to maintain this state of romantic love amid the constant demands of modern life, especially with the added complexity of a child who has special needs?

Marriage has changed. The relatively new term, "starter marriage," that's often used to describe a marriage in your twenties makes me wonder: Is it possible anymore to commit till death do you part?

Matrimony requires a delicate balance, a gentle energy, and a powerful torrent of devotion that is strong, and yet easily destroyed.

What if neither of you can point the finger of blame for disconnecting? What if fatigue, stress, and financial worries were the only bad guys in this picture? "Fault" or not, most marriages encounter a point when the matrimonial grim reaper comes calling and threatens to relegate your union to the bone-yards of failure.

What if our financial worries were blessings in disguise? If we'd had oodles of money, it's likely one or both of us would have ended our loneliness in search of that spine-tingling state of newness. Should Marc and I seriously consider parting ways? How would we navigate this pivotal moment of choice?

The waters of change often seem murkiest before settling into their calmer, more pristine state. If only it could happen without pain. What if we could approach this inevitable, defining marital moment with only love and compassion to guide us through the storm?

I thought back to our friends' ugly divorce. Being drawn into the culvert of their dramatic separation was our pivotal moment, our wake-up call. They were our last intact married friends, and we felt as though a vow-crushing virus swept through the land, leaving carnage and destruction in its path.

Somewhere during the process of trying to be honorable supporters, a line was crossed and the virus leached into our fragile environment. I could see the fire of renewed enthusiasm shimmer in Marc's eyes as the feelings of being needed triggered a deeply suppressed need of his own.

The anguish of jealousy and fear swept over me as I watched him make connections with someone I considered my friend, a woman who now saw my husband as a quick and easy way to fill the hole that had been ripped out of her heart by the destruction of *her* marriage.

I was angry, no doubt. But a much bigger part of me saw two people I cared deeply for; people who'd been hurting but were now excited about life again, if only for a brief moment. If in a similar situation, would I not seriously contemplate the options? I know I would.

What if I loved the man I'd spent the past twenty-four years with so much that seeing him come to life again actually made me happy for him? What if I was willing to let him go, simply because I felt at least one of us deserved to be happy?

But being spiritually surrendered and being authentic can be wildly opposing energies. I was worried I'd go dark and dive back into the pit of negativity that nearly drowned me only two years earlier. Did I want to mess this all up now? Did I want to undo all the good that had finally returned to our lives? No. I knew my heart and soul would survive, no matter the outcome. I knew my reaction to this moment would shape my future, a future I had been successfully improving upon daily.

This was no time to Muggle-out and get caught up in fear. The fear was there, but did I need to act on my fear, or could I act on the other emotion also within me – the love I had for this man whom I'd devoted myself to for so long? If I could act with love for both of the people who seemed to be ripping out my heart, there could only be the best possible outcome. I had to believe this.

As you can imagine, writing about this moment is a delicate matter, one that I have given much thought to and will do my best to describe – without describing. So, with much anguish and a lot of uncertainty, going on the Alaskan cruise essentially opened the door for my husband to explore his feelings for this other woman while I was away. These feelings would go as far as a kiss and would inevitably force us to determine, finally, what we wanted for our marriage.

Could we actually separate? Did we want a divided life for us, for our children? Did we want to be another statistic? The choice seemed obvious. I wouldn't be able to continue another day in a relationship that no longer functioned. If I was going to do this, we needed to make a commitment to one another again, to renew our union. Or, we would have to part. We had no middle ground anymore. If our marriage was to survive, we needed to identify our needs, communicate them skillfully, and make our marriage a priority. I wasn't getting any younger and was open to the reality that perhaps a fresh start with someone new would be my ultimate destiny.

Somewhere in the middle of all this turmoil, we agreed to each make a *What I Need to Be Happy* list. We worked on our lists together to the best of our abilities, like a vision board for our marriage. If we could identify the problems, we should be able to find solutions. We had survived so much since Emma's diagnosis; we had to at least try.

As you might guess, the top items on Marc's list included a new career direction and better financial stability. For me, I wanted more opportunities for a full night's sleep.

This dramatic turn of events forced us to finally confront one another and communicate our needs, relating in a way we hadn't for years.

As a team again, united in a common goal, we began pouring our energy back into our marriage – a marriage that, much to our surprise, stayed intact; a marriage I can say became stronger than either of us expected; a marriage I will never again take for granted, because the Grim Reaper still lurks in the shadows searching for his next weary couple.

But it won't be us this time, and for that I'm grateful.

So what about the other woman you may wonder... *So what,* indeed.

Perhaps I may become enlightened enough to thank her some day.

Perhaps.

Chapter 23

A Cure for Emma

September 2009

WE'D NEVER TRAVELED TO BOSTON before. I loved the clean, healthy feel of the city. Everywhere we looked people were jogging, biking, or rowing down the Charles River.

Our taxi driver worked his way through Williams Tunnel, beneath the bustling Boston Harbor, as we headed for the economy hotel we'd booked four months earlier. I looked at Emma, who was both nervous and excited about this trip. She loves hanging out with me, just us girls and was eager to overcome her fear of flying, even if it meant enduring blood tests once we landed. It's ironic and a big, fat bummer to be a diabetic who's petrified of needles. So we upped the ante for her eleventh birthday and agreed to buy her a laptop, provided she'd commit to putting up with Dr. Faustman's groundbreaking blood tests.

In reality, Dr. Faustman is an angel in a lab coat, a scientist at Massachusetts General Hospital in Boston. Dr. Faustman has cured type 1 diabetes in mice and is currently working on reproducing her results with humans. Her studies are the most promising and logical approach I've seen yet, and that's why we had made the trek to meet her almost four years after Emma's diagnosis.

I first received information about Dr. Faustman's work shortly after Emma and I aggressively began an organic, alkaline diet as outlined in books by Dr. Gabriel Cousins, Dr. Robert Young, and Hallelujah Acres, to name a few. These diets had been effective in reversing type 2 diabetes, as well as showing improvements for better control with type 1. We did in fact see an improvement in Emma's A1C (a test that measures how much glucose has been sticking to blood cells over the past three months.) However, I was wary when some of these sources publicized an actual *cure* for Type 1 diabetes. Following my policy to keep an open mind for possible options, I ventured down this path with cautious enthusiasm.

I have since learned that the topic of diet is a tar-pit of sticky goo when it comes to discussions within the diabetes community, especially regarding the differences between type 1 diabetes and type 2. As I'm not an expert on type 2, I will mostly stick to what I know about type 1. Diet is perhaps the largest area of misinformation T1's face in their day-to-day dealings. We still have family members who suggest to Emma that she should have an orange instead of a cookie, "because of her condition."

Let's just clear the air right now on that one and say: When you have type 1 diabetes, you no longer make enough insulin to live. This is not like Great Grandma Gerti with type 2, who manages her "sugar diabetes" by skipping dessert.

The cause of type 1 diabetes has nothing to do with eating too much sugar. With type 1, the immune system literally kills the cells that make insulin. Emma cannot eat an orange, OR a cookie without giving herself enough insulin to cover the carbs (which is the same amount when eating either snack), to allow the glucose to enter her cells. In fact, without insulin, she could go a whole day without eating anything at all, and still go into life threatening DKA because the body itself requires insulin just to keep organs and muscles working. And, while I'm at it, there are no levels of severity to type 1 diabetes, no "good kind of type 1" versus a "bad kind." It doesn't get any worse than *not making insulin*, and that's what sets type 1 apart from type 2. What matters the most in type 1 is how well you can manage your job of being a pancreas. This job is even more difficult with diabetics who are "brittle," meaning they're extra sensitive to adjustments with food and insulin.

A type 1 diabetic on an insulin pump can eat whatever they like, whenever they like, because they can and must bolus insulin for their food right there on the spot, similar to what a normal pancreas would do. No need to turn down holiday desserts or birthday cakes just because you have type 1. You simply need to know how much insulin to give yourself. Type 1 diabetics can live a normal life and participate in eating as any non-diabetic would, as long as an adequate amount of insulin is given to cover the carbs.

Now for the logic to this. Whether you have type 1 diabetes or you don't, we should all eat a healthy diet. When our family implemented the tips and vitamins learned from the above mentioned books, along with regular exercise, Emma's A1C's were better and her insulin requirements went down. These are highly desirable effects – especially when you're diabetic – but for us, it was not a cure.

It's no secret that a healthy lifestyle helps prevent long-term damage that can happen with unhealthy choices and poor blood sugar control. At the earliest stages of this disease, I suspect diet could also aid in preserving remaining beta cells and possibly even help with regeneration. I sincerely look forward to collaboration within the scientific community on the possibility of using diet to prolong the honeymoon phase.

Meanwhile, what does it all mean? For me, it means I do my best to allow Emma to be a kid, to eat desserts and roast a marshmallow with the rest of her class on a school camping trip. But I prefer she eat as healthy as possible. That's why I provide nutritious dessert options and snacks for everyone. Searching for balance in the extremes seems to be my constant goal.

The end result of my discoveries with food has revealed many benefits toward a healthier future. But I feel diet is only a puzzle piece in the big picture of this complex disease. After making a serious attempt at learning to eat like gourmet rabbits, we have since decided to continue a well-balanced diet, with most of our meals consisting of 60 percent plant source, alkaline ingredients.

This is when we finally decided to put our faith in the principles of quantum physics. If we can create our experiences in life with the thoughts we choose, then why not create the kind of cure that best suits us? Therefore, we declared to the universe that we wanted a cure that was easy, painless, affordable, simple, effective, and safe for the patient. We envisioned a cure that could be available to every person with type 1 diabetes and decided that until that option presented itself to us, we would forget about this whole healing T1 quest and enjoy our lives, because there was so much in life to enjoy.

That's when the email from Margaret arrived. An old colleague of Marc's, whose daughter was recently diagnosed with type 1. She wondered if we'd heard of a potential cure for diabetes through Boston, via Harvard Medical School. She had attached several riveting newsletters with contact information.

I sat in near disbelief as I read every word. You would think I'd be jaded to this sort of thing by then – random, too-good-to-be-true promises. I did wonder at first if this one was some kind of joke. I'd followed many promising potential cures, starting with every natural therapy modality known to man (which yielded much improved health, but no cure). I had investigated all scientific advancements, including...

- Pancreas Transplants: Last resort procedure, mostly for adults in need of a kidney transplant requiring immune suppressing drugs.
- Artificial Pancreas: Cool prototype technology, and when approved this will definitely help provide stable blood sugars for both T1 and T2. It could also play a critical role in preserving delicate transplanted islets or regeneration cells. But an artificial pancreas would not be a cure.

- Smart Insulin: Another fabulous idea, and I'd jump at the opportunity to use it for Emma should the insulin make it through the trial phases. It would also be great for type 2, but it's not available yet and would not be the cure.
- Stem Cell Research: Can create new islet cells, but still vulnerable to killer-T cell attack.
- Cell Encapsulation: Fingers are crossed on this one, great idea for protecting transplanted cells, still working out the bugs, lots of potential here.
- Islet Cell Transplants: Unfortunately, immune suppressing drugs are still the obstacle to this approach, especially for children. This is where encapsulation or protective bioengineered devices could come into play, but for now we're still left short of the miracle we've been seeking. Until someone can figure out how to eliminate the cause of T1 – the killer-T cells – I believe the solution to this problem will continue to elude us.

I forced my deflating thoughts to the side and eagerly picked up the phone to call Dr. Faustman's lab myself. It *was* real; Dr. Faustman did exist. This was good!

The kind, intelligent assistant who answered the phone was excited and enthusiastic about their work. Within a half hour of receiving the hopeful e-mail, which seemed to divinely land in my inbox, we had our arrangements set to travel to Boston.

~ ~ ~ ~

Our taxi driver finally found our hotel through the dark alleys of the waterfront. We checked in, and after three different card keys, we managed to gain access to our room. Apparently we were spoiled with our Hilton Head condo because it only took a few minutes to realize why economy rooms are ... well ... economy. After an uncomfortable night, a cold shower, and no available food, we got on the phone in search of a Marriot hotel, which has never let us down. We came across a Marriot on 777 Memorial Drive, the phone number also ending with 7777.

"This sounds like we'll do much better with all the 7's, Em. What do you think?" I asked as she gingerly sat down on the bed, her eyes on the lookout for nasty stains.

"Yes, let's go. Now!"

Emma and I have always liked the number 7. It has a good feel to us. The Marriot even gave us a special discount for being patients at Mass General. Within a couple of hours we'd checked into our glorious Marriot room #1117 and danced with joy over the much-improved accommodations. Our view of the river was charming.

Over the next two days our taxi rides cost $7.75 each time. Then, after taking a ferry to the aquarium one day and hiking to Bunker Hill on our final day, we noticed yet again more 7's. Bunker Hill, the scene of a battle fought on June 7, 1775, revealed a definite trend. It was becoming hilarious how often we saw the number 7, the very number I chose as a post office box shortly after Emma was diagnosed. This continued for our entire trip. Emma's AIC blood test was 7. The flight numbers on our plane tickets were 7775 and flight 7777. Wow! We had something cool going on with this whole number thing. I would later ask some of my spiritual friends if they knew what 7 could mean and received the following possibilities: *The number 7 can mean a spiritual journey, filled with loyalty and love. A time of transition and change. A time to do more than read or study, but to actually live and practice your truth.* To me, that sounded just right.

Meeting Dr. Faustman was, of course, the main reason for our trip. She did not disappoint us with her gentle, friendly manner and passion for her work. She laughed and smiled with Emma as she drew Emma's blood and discussed all the possibilities of her research with us. All the while, my intuitive nudge from within kept telling me: *This is it! She's the one.*

To describe her work briefly, a vaccine has been around since 1921 for tuberculosis and is also used to treat bladder cancer. This vaccine, called Bacillus Calmette-Guérin (or BCG) is inexpensive and now known to eliminate the dreaded killer-T cells responsible for attacking the insulin-producing cells of the pancreas. In mice, when these killer-T cells are eliminated, the pancreas regenerates quickly, and supplemental insulin is no longer required.

The goal of phase II of human clinical trials with BCG, which should begin as soon as they've raised enough money, (hopefully soon), will be to figure out what dosages are needed for the best results. The obstacles are similar to the challenge when insulin was discovered. Too little insulin garnered nothing. Too much insulin could cause death. So they're working out these details with BCG using a highly specialized test to count the killer-T cells in each patient. These numbers will help determine the dosage required for each individual.

BCG is only a treatment, however, and only for type 1 patients, because type 2 does not involve the release of killer-T cells. Eliminating the cause of beta cell destruction is, in my opinion, the foundation for any potential cure, which is why this particular research has me so excited.

Imagine the possibilities if BCG lives up to its potential, making insulin management and nighttime blood sugar checks outdated. Every patient would be different, so it's hard to say definitively, but a T1 diabetic might only require a needle once a month to keep the killer-T cells at bay, providing total freedom from the burdens of diabetes.

Finally getting a glimpse of what we have prayed for feels surreal. This whole Law of Attraction thing is not as easy as it looks. I have found that focusing too hard on trying to fix a problem can actually embolden the very thing I don't want. Only when I release my desires and expectations with faith do good things seem to unfold naturally. The process is kind of like watching for a parcel in the mail: you can go to the mailbox every day and it won't be there. But sure enough, the day you forget to check, your package arrives.

I have no way of knowing if Dr. Faustman's work will turn out to be what we asked for, but I have a great feeling about it, and I've now learned to trust my gut feelings. The fact that Dr. Faustman managed to show, within the highly rigid scientific community, that beta cells *can* regenerate is most impressive.

At this point I can't ignore the topic of vaccines, because I suspect it's possible the multiple injections we subjected Emma to before our unfortunate vacation may have overburdened her immune system. Over the years almost everything has been blamed for causing T1D, including cow's milk, early introduction of cereal, absence of breast feeding, too much hygiene, and too many vaccinations. The truth is, I will probably never know what triggered T1 in Emma, but the timing makes me suspect vaccinations.

I'm not saying vaccines are necessarily bad; they have created many wonderful outcomes. Smallpox, for example, was responsible for an estimated 400 million deaths during the 20th century alone. The World Health Organization (WHO) estimated 15 million people contracted smallpox and two million died as recently as 1967. After successful vaccination campaigns, the WHO certified the eradication of smallpox on December 9, 1979. To this day, smallpox is the only human infectious disease we have eradicated.

I stand by the fact that I'm not against vaccinations. Polio, mumps, measles, and rubella vaccines are all important. I merely suggest that the schedules and amounts to which we subject our children have gotten out of control. Let's go back to the 1989 U.S. schedule when the number of shots was only ten. What happened after 1990 when vaccines for our children tripled? Autism went through the roof and autoimmune diseases became epidemic. Do we truly need all these vaccinations, all at once, starting on the second day of life no less? Logic and common sense could prevent overburdening our children's bodies' during the most delicate and crucial times for their developing immune systems. Perhaps we could reverse the unwanted trends we are seeing in our children's health if we go back to a more reasonable immunization schedule. My grandfather used to say, "Too much of anything is never good." I think vaccination is a perfect example.

That's my mom-vent for the day, and unfortunately not something the medical establishment supports.

Wow. What an interesting position I find myself in. Could the very thing I suspect contributed to Emma's disease be the hero to cure it? Can one actually find balance in a world with so many extremes? I certainly hope so. I guess this is a good reminder for me to…*just stay open*. I hope to never stray too far to one side over another.

As we reached cruising altitude on #7777 flight home, I gazed past the wing and into the clouds and found myself slipping into a daydream of sorts. Could this be the beginning of a new life for us, a new life for so many others? What *would* our lives be like?

~~~~

The waves pull in toward the shore, their white, frothy peaks caressing my feet. The cool water feels so good after a long walk along the firm sand. Emma calls to me as she reaches down to pick up yet another perfect shell for her collection. Will races over to compare her find with his. This is our favorite strip of beach on Hilton Head. The prime shell treasure cove is a long walk, but worth every minute of effort.

The wind is gentle and the billowing clouds roll over the horizon. I notice a few fishing boats out for an early evening troll and decide it must be time for dinner. Marc will be back from his golf game soon, and we can all sit on the patio on this perfect evening.

As I grip the sand beneath my toes, I see a flash of the last time we were here. How easy it is now to forget all the extra concerns I once harbored for even such a simple excursion. It's okay if Will wants the last juice box – no more bottles of insulin, lancets, or infusion sites. I'm well rested, *finally*! I'm eagerly the first one up
~~~~

each morning, leaving me time to sneak out for a jog along this glorious beach above the glow of the sunrise.

I see both Emma and Will free from limitation as they stroll ahead of me, unencumbered by fear as they go out into this magnificent world. They know miracles are real and will forever live knowing and sharing this truth. I see Marc and myself free to live in our own truths, no longer letting the burden of worry consume us, believing in the greater good of all things, no matter the path. What a sense of completion and accomplishment. What a healing ripple to be felt by the rest of the world.

~ ~ ~ ~

Sure. This may have been only a daydream, but it seemed like a vision to me. I finally saw the purpose in trying to write our story: to bring awareness to the role we humans play in changing our experience, and to send our desire to cure T1 diabetes out into the universe.

The very action of reading this book will put into motion the potential for this to happen, technically speaking, like an experiment of intention. To help facilitate this goal, we will pledge a percentage of every book sold toward Dr. Faustman's research.

~ ~ ~ ~

I'm no one special, just an average everyday person like most people I know. I am grateful for my life and for the awareness of a much bigger picture than myself.

As I've worked on my crying inner child, I have helped ease the suffering of all the crying children in the world.

As I've worked to heal my body, I have helped to heal the earth and sea.

As I've worked to solve conflicts with the people within my life, I have paved the way for solving global conflicts, for peace.

And as I cure my limiting beliefs and negative thoughts, I allow room for cures to disease and illness.

Imagine if we could all work on these aspects of our lives.

Exciting times lie ahead as my children enter into a new age of clarity about the connections we share with all things. I believe as light continues to shine into the darkest of corners, as we learn to view our lives as a significant contribution to the whole of humanity, and as we treat ourselves as the radiant, loving, compassionate, powerful energy beings we are, there will no longer be room for darkness. We will finally realize there is no such thing as being special, because we are *all* special. And when everyone is special, no one person can stand out alone from the rest.

I'm no one special... and I *can* save the world.

Chapter 24

Ruby Slippers

Emma's Grade Six Class Speech Competition ~ February 2010

DO YOU BELIEVE IN MIRACLES? Picture a small woman lifting a car off the ground to rescue her trapped child after a horrible car accident. How can a one-hundred-thirty pound woman lift a thousand-pound car?

At that moment, in the craziness of an accident, all that matters to the mom is saving her child. The logic that says there is no way she should be able to lift a car doesn't even enter her mind. The only intention she has is to get her child to safety!

How is it then, that some people can defy what we believe to be possible and experience a miracle?

Ladies and gentlemen, boys and girls, and honorable judges, perhaps it can be explained with some basic physics. Quantum physics, that is.

Quantum physicists have been conducting experiments ever since Albert Einstein concluded that everything in the universe is made of energy – his formula for this being $E=MC^2$. That means the tables in our classrooms are energy, our bodies are energy, even a marshmallow is energy.

Quantum physicists have also discovered that our very thoughts emit energy, which can determine the outcome of experiments. And the best thing about energy is that it is connected to the energy of the whole universe, like a big energy spider web. This means my personal energy field can affect, on some level, the energy of everything in existence. We are all connected!

Imagine then, if I think a positive thought, it can be felt on some level, *by you*. Scientifically speaking, our thoughts are like our very own connection to everything. This is possibly the most incredible knowledge in the whole universe, a miracle that is available to everyone, including the mother who can lift the car off her child. Because, in that moment, her focus is so pure she can tap into limitless possibilities and become superhuman. She is no longer bound by skeptical logic.

Quantum physics says that there are many possible outcomes of reality at any given moment. If we are all connected to the energy of the universe, then anything should be possible. Unfortunately, most of us haven't developed that part of our awareness just yet. It's likely hidden in one of the huge, unused sections of our brains, waiting to be tapped into. It's something I think kids seem to be more open to, but lose as we grow up.

I feel that kids have a leg up on most grown-ups when it comes to miracles, because it's still easy for us to believe in anything. Our thoughts are usually always focused on good feelings – not because our parents try to teach us this, but because it's standard equipment with kids. I have type 1 diabetes, and I believe that I'll be cured. I may be just a kid, but I think that with a little help from the principles of quantum physics, I can attract a way to create a cure for myself and the millions who are out there, like me – if for no other reason, than because I want to.

One way to help us connect to the limitless nature of the universe would be to pay attention to the words we all use every day. Are we affirming what we want most of the time, or are we saying what we don't want more often?

There are old nursery rhymes and prayers out there that never made much sense to me, like Rock-a-bye Baby. The words: "On the treetop, when the wind blows, the cradle will rock, when the bough breaks, the cradle will fall, and down will come baby, cradle and all..." What kind of positive thoughts are those before going to bed?

Then there is the prayer: "Now I lay me down to sleep, I pray to God my soul to keep. If I die before I wake, I pray to God my soul to take."

I see the original purpose in this prayer, but I definitely don't want to think about dying in my sleep before I wake up! Maybe it's time to update the words we use in our lives just a little. How about something like this instead:

As we prepare to go to sleep,
We pray to the universe our dreams to seek.
While we soar as formless light,
We feel compassion for the world tonight.

When we wake, we'll be renewed.
Strong, healthy and vibrant, too.
Thank you, God, for everything under the sun,
for we know in our hearts that we are all one.

Thank you for guidance as type 1 diabetes is cured.
We are grateful for this opportunity and
eagerly share it with the rest of the world.
Amen.

That makes me feel good before going to bed; and when I feel good I know I'm helping the whole world to feel good, scientifically speaking.

Isn't it great that science can prove what we already know in our hearts, that miracles can simply result from a choice!

To me, quantum physics equals the power of our intentions. Like a pair of *Magical Ruby Slippers* on our feet that someone forgot to tell us how to use.

I believe in miracles. Do you?

Emma

Epilogue

April 2010

MOJO SITS QUIETLY BY THE FIRE as snow gently falls on our sleepy little town. Just when we thought winter was over, Mother Nature decides to add one last chilling reminder to keep our snow tires on until May. You gotta love Canada.

My angelfish swim about happily, completely unaware of the radical weather outside my window. Their view is unchanged, exactly the way they like it.

Mojo stretches out, face up to take in the full heat of what should be one of our last fires of the season, pulling her paws over her head and curiously tilting her furry little chin. From that position she can see her angelfish to the left and her typing human to the right. She has one of those undeniable looks on her face as she glances toward me, still upside down, the: it-doesn't-get-any-better-than-this look.

"You're right, Mojo ... it really doesn't get any better than this," I respond.

Indeed, I often sit still in silent moments like these and close my eyes, listening to the resonance of life that surrounds me – my life. Sometimes it may be the giggles of my children in the other room, or the chirp of a bird in a tree by my window. Right now, it's the sloshing sound fresh snow makes as cars drive past.

I have many plans for the future, including our next trip to Boston to see Dr. Faustman. As excited as I am about the adventures that lie ahead and the possibilities for Emma's future without diabetes, I'm equally thrilled by the journey in front of me and by the incredible beauty that surrounds me every day. I like nothing better than snuggling in front of that fire on a cold day with a good book to read, or in today's case, a good book to write.

I look back at Mojo and recall the first morning I came here to type my thoughts. She was so small then, fitting on my lap without interfering with the pitter-patter of my fingers along the keyboard, as long as she wasn't chasing the mouse marker on my screen.

Now, three years later she's matured and mellowed from a rambunctious, tree-climbing kitten, and it feels as though I've grown and matured right along with her. If I hadn't been journaling the events of the past few years, would I even have noticed all the changes we've experienced? Would I appreciate how grateful I am to still live in my treasured home? Would I have seen how our last Hilton Head vacation prompted the beginning of the perfect career for Marc? As I write these words, Marc now sits in his home office above our garage preparing for his first bag of quality wood pellets to come off the line.

This change didn't happen overnight. Marc and his partners worked hard over the past year to bring this dream to fruition. Nonetheless, he is now a proud new entrepreneur and owner of a bioenergy company. And here *we* are, a dedicated team, working together from home toward our goals. Having Marc around has been an adjustment; a good adjustment.

Living as a spiritual being in this human world is quite an adjustment as well. One of my favorite stories that brought this concept into perspective for me is a piece I read from the Sufi poet, Rumi. This story is an Arab tale of a man in the thirteenth century who seeks advice from a wise old man.

"I believe God is watching over me," he says. "So if I tie up my camel at night, I'm afraid it will mean I don't have enough faith in

God. But if I don't tie up my camel and it runs away, I'll feel like a fool. I don't know what to do."

To which the wise man replies:

"Trust in God – AND tie up your camel!"

If I've learned anything to offer my children, it is this: Always be willing to do the work that needs to be done, and remain confident that, when the time is right, your prayers will always be answered. The promise of your dreams will forever be available to you, provided you *remain open* to receive them, in divine balance.

Mojo gets up with a long stretch and walks towards the phone. She sits staring at it, as though the telephone is about to do a trick of some kind.

"What is it, Mojo?"

Before I can give it a second thought, the phone rings.

I get up to check the call display. It's my mother. Sheesh, here comes the bi-yearly phone call.

"Crap, Mojo! I don't think I'm up for this one." She rubs on my leg and throws one of those irresistible purr-meows at me.

"Brrrrreoowww."

"Oh no ... no, no, no, don't pull that. I'm having such a nice quiet morning; I don't need to spoil it.

"Brrrrreoowww."

"I know, I know. I *can* do it. I just don't know if I want to."

I take advantage of two more rings as I breathe in the peace around me. I know in my heart I am greater than the fear sneaking up inside me at the mere thought of picking up the phone. I'm safe and secure, and besides, I still haven't found out why she liked the name Ann.

I reach for the phone with a hopeful heart.

Just stay open ... Just stay open...

Type 1 Diabetes and Dr. Denise Faustman

*TYPE 1 DIABETES is one of the most common endocrine and metabolic conditions in childhood. The incidence is rapidly increasing, especially among the youngest children. Insulin-treatment, although lifesaving, requires lifelong commitment and is painful, time-consuming, and interferes with daily life. Managing this disease calls for self-discipline and adherence to a balanced diet. Access to self-care tools and insulin is limited in many countries, especially for less privileged families, which may lead to severe handicaps and early death in diabetic children.

Many children and adolescents are unable to emotionally cope with their condition.

Diabetes can cause embarrassment, resulting in discrimination and limiting social relationships. This invisible disease may impact school performance, family functioning, and lead to family disruption and divorce. Parents experience a financial burden and may have to reduce their working hours or give up work entirely to care for their child. The financial burden may be aggravated by the costs of new treatment and monitoring modalities, such as insulin pumps and continuous, real-time glucose monitoring devices.

*International Diabetes Federation, *IDF Diabetes Atlas*, fourth edition. Diabetes in the Young: a Global Perspective.

Unsatisfactory metabolic control in children can result in stunted growth and exposure to both severe hypoglycaemia and chronic hyperglycaemia, which can adversely affect neurological development. Although the cumulative incidence of diabetic nephropathy (kidney disease) has fallen over the last few decades in dedicated centers, this trend is by no means universal. Recent observations have shown that children who avoid microvascular complications may still face the prospect of accelerated atherosclerosis.

Evidence tells us the incidence of childhood onset type 1 diabetes is increasing in many countries. Overall, the annual increase is estimated around 3 percent. Evidence also suggests that, in relative terms, these increases are greatest in young children.

In 2010, 75,800 children under the age of fourteen were diagnosed with type 1. That was 207 children per day, or one new case every seven minutes!

Hundreds of T1 cure warriors are working to solve the puzzle of type 1 diabetes and find a cure. Two of the most respected organizations are the Juvenile Diabetes Research Foundation (The leading fund raising entity in the world), which raised billions of dollars over the past forty years, and The Diabetes Research Institute in Miami, Florida, armed with many of the world's top scientists dedicated to curing T1.

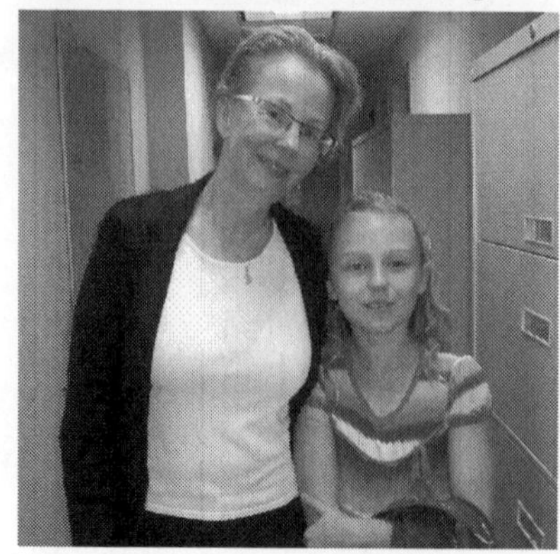
Dr. Faustman (left)
Emma Colvin (right)

My intention for this book is to support one Cure Warrior from MGH who stands out among her peers: Doctor Denise L. Faustman, who has worked in the field of autoimmunity for over fifteen years and made key discoveries regarding the role of MHC Class I antigen presentation in immunity. After completing her internship, residency, and fellowships in Internal Medicine and Endocrinology at the Massachusetts General Hospital, Dr. Faustman became an independent investigator at the MGH and Harvard Medical School in 1987. Since then, she has cured mice of type 1 diabetes by stopping the assault of killer-T cells upon pancreatic islet cells. Phase I of human clinical trials concluded in 2010 with excellent results, and phase II will begin as soon as sufficient funds have been raised.

Dr Faustman's honors in recent years include:

- 2006: Women in Science Award, American Medical Women's Association and Wyeth Pharmaceutical Company. This award is given to a woman physician who has made exceptional contributions to medical science through basic science publications and leadership in the field.
- 2005: Oprah Achievement Award, Top Health Breakthrough by a Female Scientist.
- 2003: National Institutes of Health and the National Library of Medicine's "Changing the Face of Medicine" award. Dr. Faustman was one of 300 American physicians honored for achievement in medicine, past and present.

Dr. Faustman's research depends on donations from the public. Business icon Lee Iacocca lost his wife to diabetic complications at the age of fifty-seven. He established The Iacocca Foundation twenty years ago and pledged to find a cure within his lifetime. Iacocca is so confident in Dr. Faustman's approach that he committed all the foundation's resources, plus a million dollars of his own money, to Dr. Faustman. But that isn't enough. Scientific trials cost time and money; millions of dollars are needed to complete the final two phases of this trial.

A Cure for Emma will donate a portion of the book's profits to Dr. Faustman's cutting-edge research. We invite you to donate as well. Learn more about the study on Dr. Faustman's web page: www.faustmanlab.org

To make a donation today, please go to: https://give.massgeneral.org/SSLPage.aspx?pid=388

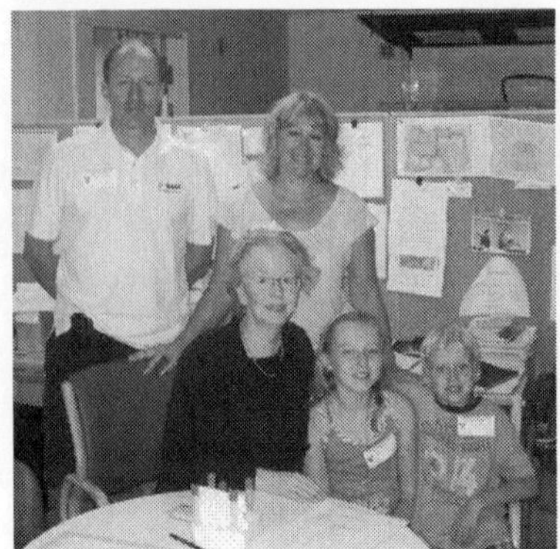

The Colvin Family with
Dr. Faustman

On June 26th 2011, Dr. Faustman attended the scientific meetings of the American Diabetes Association (ADA), where she presented additional results from the Phase I human clinical trial. This trial tested BCG vaccination as a treatment for advanced type 1 diabetes. The data showed BCG treatment, or similar therapy, has potential to briefly get the pancreas working, even in people who've had type 1 diabetes for many years.

Data from the Phase I study show that BCG treatment:

- eliminated disease-causing T cells that attack the pancreas,
- increased the number of beneficial regulatory T cells (Tregs),
- restored the ability of the pancreas to secrete insulin for a time.

Notably, the study participants had been living with type 1 diabetes for an average of 15 years.

These results are strengthened by data from one placebo-treated patient who unexpectedly developed Epstein-Barr virus (EBV) infection after the study began, yet experienced the same beneficial effects as those who were treated with BCG. Like BCG vaccination, Epstein-Barr infection boosts the level of tumor necrosis factor (TNF) in the body, which researchers believe is the mechanism through which BCG treatment benefits human type 1 diabetes.

Phase I is the earliest stage of clinical testing, so it's too soon to throw away our insulin needles, but these exciting results indicate the pancreas may regenerate after BCG treatment. The next step is a Phase II study.

Thanks to the leadership role of the Iacocca Foundation, MGH has reached $8.5 million in funding for Phase II. This means Phase II work can begin. Please make a donation to help sustain the momentum so the foundation can meet their total need of $25 million to complete Phase II over the next three years.

From the Author

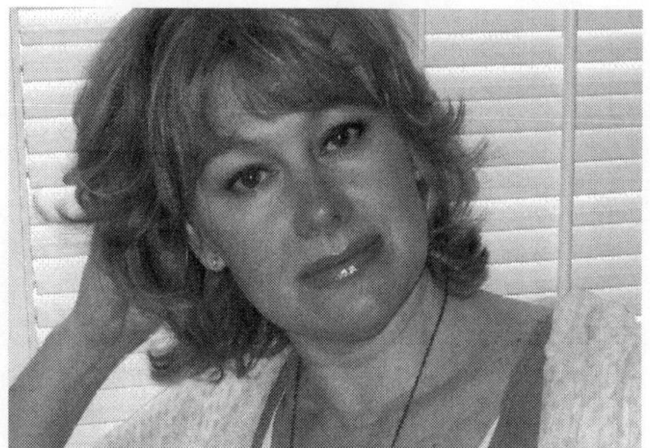

Julie Colvin

DURING FOURTEEN YEARS as a Registered Diagnostic Medical Sonographer, I acquired a vast knowledge of the body and its organ systems. Not until disease struck my family did I become aware of a larger picture of health – one that involved natural holistic approaches, self-empowerment, and the thoughts we choose to think.

I have since been dedicated to learning healing modalities that involve the dynamics of what we are made of – *Energy*. And what fuels that energy – *Our Beliefs*. My ultimate motivation has been my family and our goal to achieve a healthy balance of body, mind, and spirit.

I have learned many different natural therapy modalities, including VoiceBio analysis, reflexology, spiritual psychology, energy healing facilitation, quantum touch, and emotional freedom techniques. I love to mix this natural wisdom with my base of medical awareness. I find it keeps me grounded while I navigate between these two worlds.

Beautiful northern Ontario, Canada is the place I call home, shared with my husband and two incredible children. I look forward to a lifetime of learning and an opportunity to share my experiences with others embarking on a journey to better health.

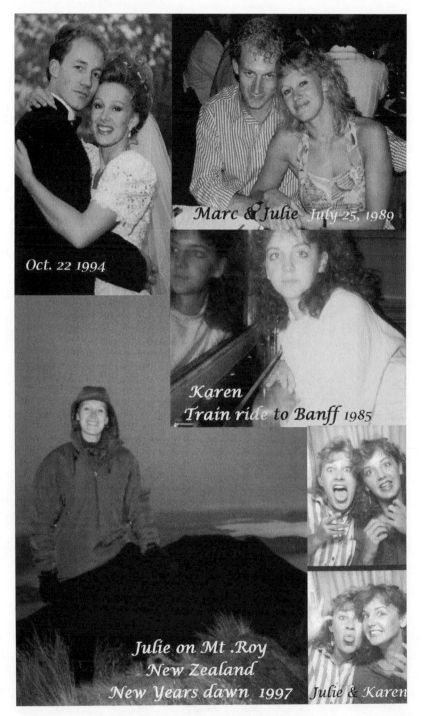
Oct. 22 1994
Marc & Julie July 25, 1989
Karen
Train ride to Banff 1985
Julie on Mt .Roy
New Zealand
New Years dawn 1997
Julie & Karen

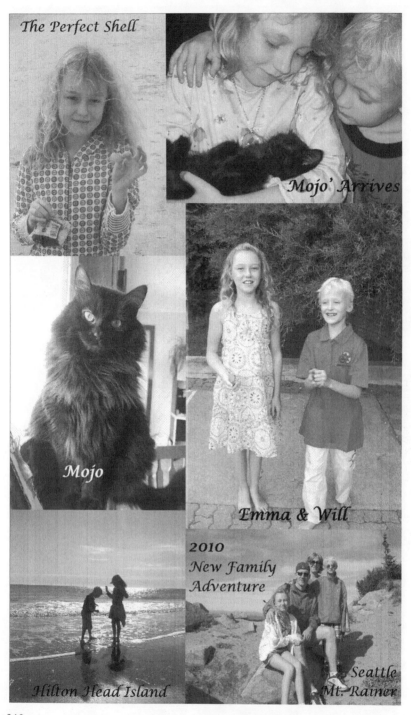
The Perfect Shell
Mojo' Arrives
Mojo
Emma & Will
Hilton Head Island
2010
New Family
Adventure
Seattle
Mt. Rainer

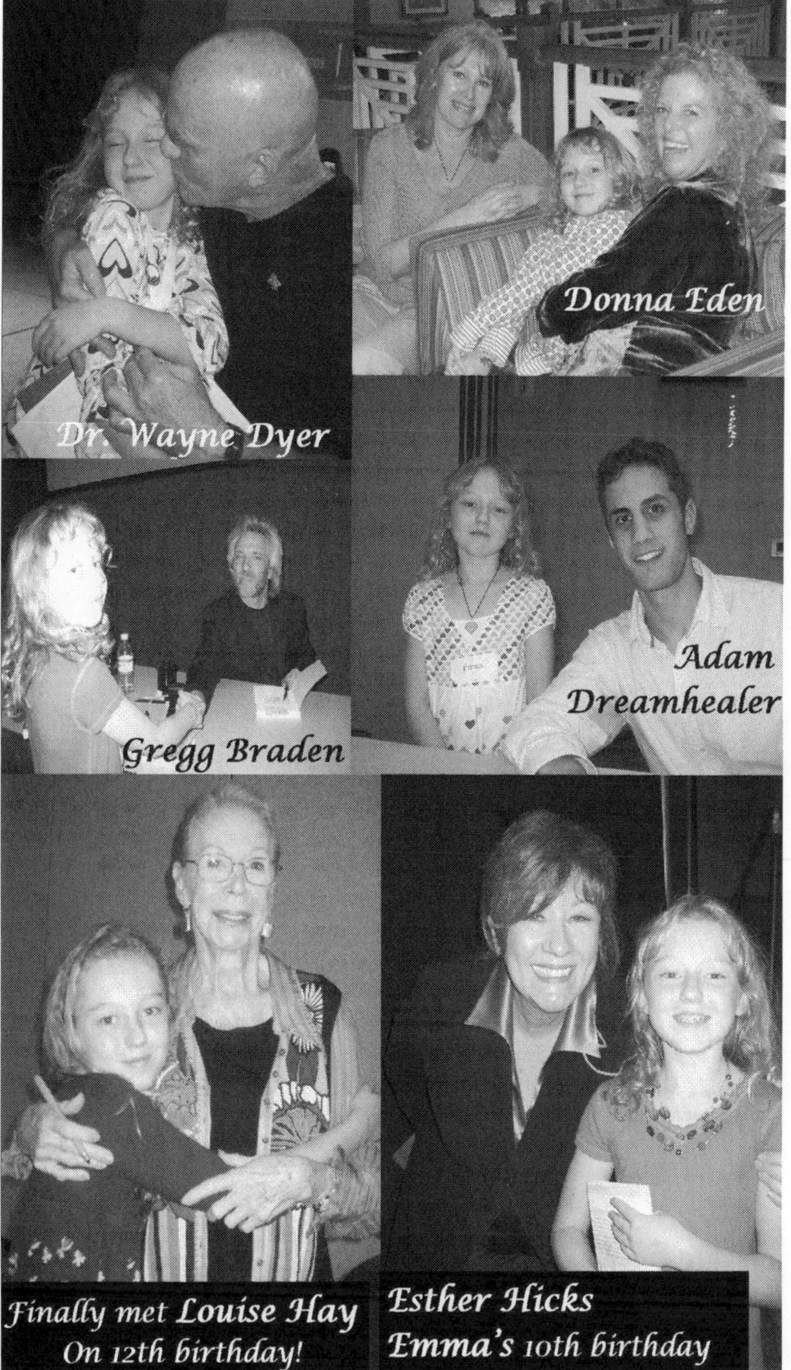
Dr. Wayne Dyer
Donna Eden
Gregg Braden
Adam
Dreamhealer
Finally met Louise Hay
On 12th birthday!
Esther Hicks
Emma's 10th birthday

Available from NorlightsPress and fine booksellers everywhere

Toll free: 888-558-4354 **Online:** www.norlightspress.com
Shipping Info: Add $2.95 - first item and $1.00 for each additional item

Name ______________________________

Address ______________________________

Daytime Phone ______________________________

E-mail ______________________________

No. Copies	Title	Price (each)	Total Cost

Subtotal	
Shipping	
Total	

Payment by (circle one):
Check Visa Mastercard Discover Am Express

Card number ______________________________ 3 digit code ________

Exp.date ____________ Signature ______________________________

Mailing Address:

762 State Road 458
Bedford IN 47421

Sign up to receive our catalogue at www.norlightspress.com

Made in the USA
Lexington, KY
22 February 2014